Diet Types and Their Impact on Lifespan

I0446843

A very short introduction from
The HealthSpan Institute

Diet Types and Their Impact on Lifespan
A Very Short Introduction from The HealthSpan Institute
  ISBN: 9798865164197

Printed in the United States of America

Contents

Introduction

Chapter 1:
The Basics of Lifespan and Diet

Chapter 2:
Mediterranean Diet

Chapter 3:
Vegan and Vegetarian Diets

Chapter 4:
Paleo Diet

Chapter 5:
Ketogenic Diet

Chapter 6:
Plant-based Whole Foods Diet

Chapter 7:
Intermittent Fasting and Caloric Restriction

Chapter 8:
Blue Zones – Lessons from the Longest Lived

Chapter 9:
The Role of Supplements and Longevity

Chapter 10:
Pitfalls of Modern Diets

Chapter 11:
Integrating Diet with Other Longevity Practices

Holistic approaches to longevity: combining diet, exercise, and mindfulness 104

Chapter 12:
Personalizing Your Dietary Approach

Recognizing individual differences in dietary needs and responses 107

Tips for experimentation and finding what works for each individual 109

Chapter 13:
Conclusion

Appendix A:
Glossary of terms

Appendix B:
Recommended reading and resources

Appendix C:
Sample meal plans and recipes for each diet type

Introduction

Background on the Importance of Diet on Overall Health and Longevity

The age-old adage "You are what you eat" holds more truth than we often give it credit for. Over the last few decades, an increasing body of scientific research has reinforced the profound influence diet has on our overall health, well-being, and longevity. More than just providing the fuel to sustain our daily activities, the foods we consume play a pivotal role in determining the quality and duration of our lives.

The Cellular Impact of Diet

At the microscopic level, every morsel of food we ingest interacts with our cells. Nutrients—whether vitamins, minerals, antioxidants, or macronutrients—impact cell behavior, integrity, and function. For example, antioxidants found in colorful fruits and vegetables combat oxidative stress, a primary driver of cellular aging. Conversely, diets high in refined sugars and unhealthy fats can lead to cellular inflammation, potentially accelerating aging processes and paving the way for chronic diseases.

Influence on Chronic Diseases

The global rise in chronic diseases such as heart disease, diabetes, and obesity underscores the urgency of understanding the diet-health relationship. Diets high in saturated fats, trans fats, and sugars have been consistently linked with these ailments. Conversely, diets rich in whole grains, lean proteins, and abundant vegetables and fruits seem to offer protective benefits. For instance, the Mediterranean diet, rooted in olive oil, fish, and fresh produce, has been correlated with reduced risks of heart disease and longer life expectancies.

Digestion and Gut Health

The influence of diet isn't limited to the cellular level or chronic disease prevention. Our gut health, which is intrinsically linked to overall well-being, is also directly affected by our dietary choices. The gut microbiome, a diverse community of bacteria residing in our intestines, thrives on a fiber-rich diet and is disrupted by excessive sugars and artificial additives. A balanced microbiome aids digestion, nutrient absorption, and even plays a role in mood regulation and immune function. Imbalances, on the other hand, have been connected to ailments ranging from irritable bowel syndrome to mental health disorders.

Brain Health and Cognitive Function

Emerging research also suggests that our diet can influence brain health and cognitive function, particularly as we age. Omega-3 fatty acids found in fish, walnuts, and flaxseeds, for example, are essential for brain cell structure and function. Diets deficient in these fats, or overloaded with unhealthy fats, may impact cognitive abilities and increase the risk of neurodegenerative diseases like Alzheimer's.

Lifespan vs. Healthspan

While longevity—how long we live—is a topic of great interest, an equally vital consideration is healthspan: the period in our lives we remain healthy and free from debilitating diseases. It's not just about adding years to our life, but life to our years. Here again, diet emerges as a major player. A balanced, nutrient-rich diet can delay the onset of age-related diseases, ensuring that we enjoy a higher quality of life for longer.

Conclusion

In essence, our dietary choices lay the foundation for our health trajectory. They can either bolster our defenses against diseases and age-related decline or undermine our well-being, leading to early aging and diminished quality of life. As we delve deeper into understanding various diets and their impact on lifespan in the subsequent chapters, it's crucial to keep in mind the overarching importance of nutrition as one of the primary levers we can control in our pursuit of a long, fulfilling life.

Brief Overview of the Various Diets Covered

As humans, we've experimented with various dietary patterns over millennia, each reflecting our cultural, geographical, and historical contexts. Modern times have seen a rise in diverse diets, driven by health concerns, environmental considerations, and ethical reasons. Here's a succinct overview of the primary diets covered in this book:

1. Mediterranean Diet

Hailing from the Mediterranean basin, this diet emphasizes fruits, vegetables, whole grains, fish, nuts, and olive oil. Characterized by its high consumption of monounsaturated fats and low intake of red meat and dairy, the Mediterranean diet has consistently been associated with heart health and longevity.

2. Vegan and Vegetarian Diets

Both diets eschew meat, though with key differences:

- **Vegan Diet:** Excludes all animal products, encompassing meat, dairy, eggs, and often honey. Rooted in concerns for animal welfare, environmental reasons, and health, this diet is rich in plant-based foods.
- **Vegetarian Diet:** While it omits meat, variations exist based on the inclusion of dairy, eggs, or both. Lacto-vegetarians consume dairy, ovo-vegetarians eat eggs, and lacto-ovo-vegetarians include both.

3. Paleo Diet

Inspired by the presumed dietary habits of our Paleolithic ancestors, the Paleo diet focuses on whole foods like lean meats, fish, fruits, vegetables, nuts, and seeds. It excludes grains, legumes, dairy, and processed foods. Advocates argue it aligns more closely with our evolutionary nutritional needs.

4. Ketogenic Diet

A high-fat, moderate-protein, and very low-carb diet, the ketogenic or "keto" diet pushes the body into ketosis. In this metabolic state, the body burns fats for fuel instead of its default energy source, carbohydrates. While often adopted for weight loss, there's growing interest in its potential longevity benefits.

5. Plant-based Whole Foods Diet

Centered around unrefined, unprocessed plant foods, this diet promotes fruits, vegetables, whole grains, legumes, seeds, and nuts. Unlike veganism, it's not strictly about avoiding animal products but emphasizes whole, minimally processed plant foods for optimal health.

6. Intermittent Fasting and Caloric Restriction

Not diets in the traditional sense, these approaches focus on when and how much to eat:

- **Intermittent Fasting (IF):** Involves cycling between periods of eating and fasting. Popular methods include the 16/8 method (16 hours of fasting followed by an 8-hour eating window) and the 5:2 method (eating normally for five days, then drastically reducing calorie intake for two).
- **Caloric Restriction:** A consistent reduction in daily caloric intake without malnutrition. Research has shown it can increase lifespan in various organisms, sparking interest in its potential benefits for humans.

7. Blue Zones Diet

Originating from regions where people live exceptionally long lives, the Blue Zones diet is diverse but centers around plant-heavy, whole-foods-based diets with moderate protein intake, often from fish. The diet is just one component, with lifestyle factors like community and regular physical activity also playing crucial roles.

Conclusion

This variety in dietary patterns reflects the vast tapestry of human experience and our evolving understanding of nutrition. Each diet offers unique benefits and considerations, with no one-size-fits-all answer. As we dive deeper into each diet's impact on lifespan, it's worth noting that individual responses to diets can vary. Thus, personalization and attentiveness to one's body are paramount. The following chapters will provide a comprehensive understanding of each diet, guiding you towards informed choices for health and longevity.

Explanation of Key Terms and Concepts

Understanding the science of aging and longevity requires a foundational grasp of certain key terms and concepts. This section elucidates these terms, offering clarity on the nuances that distinguish them.

Lifespan

Lifespan, often referred to as 'maximum lifespan', denotes the maximum number of years an individual from a particular species can live. It represents the outer limit of life for a species, given ideal circumstances. For humans, the recorded maximum lifespan is 122 years, a record held by Jeanne Calment of France. However, it's essential to note that while lifespan indicates potential longevity, it doesn't necessarily reflect the average duration most individuals of a species will live.

Life Expectancy

A more common term used in demographic studies and public health is **life expectancy**. Life expectancy represents the average number of years a newborn individual is expected to live, given the current mortality rates in a specific population. Life expectancy can vary significantly based on factors such as geography, healthcare access, socioeconomic conditions, diet, and lifestyle. For instance, a country with advanced healthcare, low levels of violence, and high standards of living will likely have a higher life expectancy than a country grappling with poverty and disease.

It's also worth noting that life expectancy can change as an individual ages. For example, life expectancy at birth might be 75 years in a particular country. However, if a person reaches the age of 60 without major health complications, their life expectancy could exceed the initial estimate due to their having bypassed many risks associated with younger ages.

Healthspan

While lifespan and life expectancy focus on the duration of life, **healthspan** concerns the quality of those years. Healthspan represents the period in an individual's life during which they remain free from chronic diseases and maintain functional abilities, both physically and mentally. It's the duration of life spent in good health, without significant illness or disability.

Imagine two individuals, both living to the age of 85. The first individual remains active, mentally sharp, and largely disease-free until the age of 80, after which they experience a brief period of decline. In contrast, the second individual begins facing chronic illnesses from the age of 60 and spends the next 25 years managing these health issues. While both have the same lifespan, the first individual has a longer healthspan.

The concept of healthspan is gaining traction in gerontology and public health because it emphasizes the quality of life, not just its duration. With advances in medical technology, it's now possible to extend life even in the presence of chronic diseases. However, the ultimate goal for many researchers and individuals is to extend the years of healthy, active life, rather than just adding more years to life.

In Summary

Understanding the nuances between lifespan, life expectancy, and healthspan is crucial when exploring the realm of human longevity. While lifespan sets the potential limits of human life and life expectancy provides an average based on current conditions, healthspan introduces the qualitative aspect, urging us to consider not just how long we live, but how well we live those years. As we delve into the impact of various diets on longevity, these concepts will serve as critical reference points, enabling a more comprehensive grasp of the subject matter.

Chapter 1:
The Basics of Lifespan and Diet

Definition and Factors Influencing Lifespan

Lifespan, the concept of the length of life from birth to death, has intrigued humans for eons. While it's straightforward to define lifespan as the total number of years an organism lives, understanding the myriad factors that influence it presents a more intricate puzzle. This section seeks to elucidate both the definition and the complex tapestry of factors that shape lifespan.

Lifespan Defined

Lifespan, in its most unvarnished form, denotes the duration of life of an organism. For humans, it's the period from birth to death. Not to be mistaken with 'life expectancy,' which is the average age a person is expected to live based on current mortality rates, lifespan represents the absolute limits of life under optimal conditions.

For humans, the maximum recorded lifespan is 122 years, a record held by Jeanne Calment of France. However, this number doesn't suggest that everyone can or will live to this age; rather, it signifies a potential given perfect circumstances.

Factors Influencing Lifespan

Lifespan doesn't hinge on a singular factor; instead, it's the result of an intricate interplay of genetics, environment, lifestyle, and even luck. Let's delve into these factors:

1. **Genetics:** Our DNA undoubtedly plays a pivotal role in determining our lifespan. Certain genes are responsible for repairing DNA, producing proteins, and managing oxidative stress – all processes integral to aging. Some individuals might possess genetic profiles that predispose them to longer lives or reduce the risk of certain age-related diseases.

2. **Environment:** The environment in which we grow, live, and age can profoundly impact our lifespan. Factors such as pollution, exposure to harmful chemicals, radiation, and even our social environment can play a part. Societal structures that support health, safety, and well-being can contribute to longer lifespans.

3. **Diet and Nutrition:** As previously discussed, what we consume can have significant implications for longevity. Nutrient-rich diets that are balanced in macronutrients and abundant in micronutrients can promote health and stave off diseases.

4. **Physical Activity:** Regular physical activity strengthens the heart, manages body weight, and reduces the risk of chronic diseases. Active individuals often have better metabolic health, muscular strength, and bone density, all of which contribute to longevity.

5. **Medical Care:** Access to quality healthcare throughout life can have a pronounced impact on lifespan. Medical interventions can prevent or manage chronic diseases, treat acute conditions, and enhance the overall quality of life.

6. **Mental and Social Well-being:** A sound mind contributes to a long life. Chronic stress, prolonged periods of depression, or extended isolation can have deleterious effects on health. Conversely, strong social connections, mental stimulation, and a positive outlook can enhance lifespan.

7. **Luck:** While it might seem less scientific, luck, or the random events in life, plays its part. Accidents, unforeseen events, or rare diseases can influence lifespan in ways that are beyond an individual's control.

8. **Behavioral Choices:** Smoking, excessive alcohol consumption, drug use, and even prolonged sun exposure without protection are choices that can reduce lifespan. Conversely, choices such as regular health check-ups, wearing seat belts, and practicing safe behaviors can extend it.

Wrapping Up

Lifespan, while definable in a single sentence, is influenced by a convoluted web of factors. Some are within our control, and some are not. While the genetic blueprint we inherit can set certain parameters, our environment, lifestyle choices, and even chance events sculpt the final outcome. As we continue to explore diet's role in influencing lifespan, it's essential to consider it as one of the many threads in this intricate tapestry of life.

The Connection Between Diet, Genetics, and Lifestyle

The quest for understanding the determinants of human health and longevity has long been a focal point of scientific inquiry. At the intersection of this research are diet, genetics, and lifestyle – three pillars that, in unison, wield significant influence over our health outcomes. Here, we explore the intricate interplay among these factors and their collective impact on our well-being.

The Role of Genetics

Genetics form the foundational blueprint of our biological being. Every cell carries a genetic code that determines various aspects of our physiology, from eye color to predispositions to certain diseases. While we inherit this genetic framework at birth and cannot change the sequence of our DNA, recent discoveries in the field of epigenetics reveal that our genes' expression can be influenced by external factors.

1. **Gene-Diet Interaction**: The burgeoning field of nutrigenomics studies the interaction between nutrition and genes. Certain foods can turn on or off specific genes. For instance, diets rich in omega-3 fatty acids might activate genes that combat inflammation.

2. **Genetic Predispositions**: Some individuals are genetically predisposed to lactose intolerance or gluten sensitivity. Recognizing and adjusting dietary intake based on genetic predispositions can greatly impact well-being.

Dietary Choices: More Than Just Fuel

Diet does more than simply provide the energy to get through the day. It delivers essential nutrients that influence bodily functions, supports growth and repair, and offers protection against diseases.

1. **Diet and Disease:** Nutritional choices can either reduce or heighten the risk of diseases. Diets high in saturated fats and sugars have been linked to heart diseases and diabetes, while those abundant in fruits, vegetables, and whole grains offer protective benefits against several chronic conditions.

2. **Micronutrients and Bodily Functions:** Essential vitamins and minerals influence countless biochemical reactions. For example, vitamin C supports immune function, and iron is pivotal for oxygen transport in the blood.

3. **Gut Health:** The food we consume directly impacts our gut microbiota. A diverse and balanced gut flora, fostered by a varied diet rich in fiber, is linked to improved digestion, immune function, and even mental health.

Lifestyle: The Broader Canvas

Lifestyle encompasses a spectrum of choices and habits beyond just diet, including physical activity, sleep, stress management, and social connections.

1. **Physical Activity and Diet:** The synergy between diet and exercise is undeniable. Proper nutrition supports physical activity by providing the necessary energy and nutrients for muscle function and recovery. Conversely, regular exercise can enhance metabolic health and influence dietary choices by regulating appetite and cravings.

2. **Stress, Sleep, and Nutrition:** Chronic stress and lack of sleep can lead to unhealthy eating habits, like binge eating or reaching for sugary, high-fat foods. A balanced diet, in turn, can promote better sleep and help manage stress by stabilizing blood sugar levels and providing essential nutrients for neurotransmitter synthesis.

3. **Social Aspects of Diet**: Our social environments shape our dietary habits. Family traditions, cultural norms, and social gatherings all influence what and how we eat. Social connections also play a pivotal role in mental well-being, which can further influence dietary choices.

The Intertwined Trio

Diet, genetics, and lifestyle are deeply interconnected. While our genes set the stage, our dietary and lifestyle choices can either amplify or mitigate genetic predispositions. The food we consume interacts with our genetic makeup, influencing gene expression, and our broader lifestyle choices, from exercise habits to sleep patterns, further modulate these interactions.

In understanding the dance among diet, genetics, and lifestyle, we recognize that health is not merely the absence of disease but a holistic state of physical, mental, and social well-being. By making informed choices in these domains, we can steer our health journey in a direction of vitality and longevity.

How Nutrition Affects the Body at the Cellular Level

The intricate ballet of life, from our most basic movements to our most profound thoughts, hinges on the health and function of our cells. These microscopic units, the building blocks of our bodies, are profoundly influenced by the nutrients we consume. Dive deep into the cellular realm, and one discovers a world where nutrition orchestrates a myriad of biochemical processes that maintain life and health.

The Cellular Landscape

Each cell in our body is a bustling metropolis of activity. From energy production in the mitochondria to protein synthesis in the ribosomes, cells are constantly working to maintain homeostasis. Central to these operations are the nutrients we derive from our food.

Macronutrients and Cellular Energy

Macronutrients – carbohydrates, proteins, and fats – are the primary dietary components that our bodies use for energy and growth.

1. **Carbohydrates:** Once ingested, carbohydrates are broken down into glucose. This glucose enters our cells and is used in the mitochondria to produce ATP, the primary energy currency of the cell, through a process called cellular respiration.

2. **Proteins:** Comprised of amino acids, proteins are vital for almost every cellular function. They form enzymes that catalyze biochemical reactions, act as structural components of cells, and play roles in cellular signaling. After consumption, dietary proteins are broken down into their constituent amino acids, which are then used by cells to synthesize the specific proteins they need.

3. **Fats:** Essential for cellular function, fats are primary components of cell membranes, providing fluidity and flexibility. They also serve as a significant energy store. When glucose is scarce, fats are broken down in the mitochondria to produce energy.

Micronutrients: Essential Cofactors and Building Blocks

Micronutrients, the vitamins and minerals we obtain from our diet, are crucial for a plethora of cellular functions, often serving as cofactors for enzymes or playing structural roles.

1. **Vitamins:** These organic compounds are vital for cellular health. For example, B vitamins often act as coenzymes in energy production, while vitamin D is essential for calcium regulation in cells.

2. **Minerals:** These inorganic nutrients play diverse roles. Calcium, for instance, is crucial for muscle cell contraction, while iron is a key component of hemoglobin, the oxygen-carrying molecule in red blood cells.

Antioxidants: Cellular Protectors

Oxidative stress, resulting from the accumulation of free radicals, can damage cellular components like DNA, proteins, and lipids. Antioxidants, nutrients like vitamin C, vitamin E, and selenium, neutralize these free radicals, protecting cells from oxidative damage and potential subsequent diseases like cancer.

Nutrient Signaling and Gene Expression

Nutrients don't just serve as fuel or building blocks; they also influence how our genes are expressed. Nutrients can activate or deactivate specific genes, influencing cellular function and health. For instance, omega-3 fatty acids can suppress genes involved in inflammation, thus providing their noted anti-inflammatory effects.

The Cellular Consequences of Malnutrition

Without proper nutrition, cells cannot function optimally. Deficiencies in specific nutrients can lead to cellular dysfunction, manifesting as fatigue, weakened immunity, or more severe diseases. For instance, a deficiency in vitamin C impairs collagen synthesis, affecting the integrity of skin and connective tissues.

In Conclusion

Nutrition's role at the cellular level is paramount. The nutrients we consume are intricately involved in almost every cellular process, from energy production to gene expression. By understanding the profound impacts of nutrition at this microscopic scale, we can better appreciate the adage that we indeed are what we eat.

Chapter 2: Mediterranean Diet

Origins and Key Components

The Mediterranean diet, often hailed as a paradigm of healthy eating, is more than just a dietary regimen; it's a reflection of a rich cultural and historical tapestry that spans several countries surrounding the Mediterranean Sea. Let's embark on a journey to understand its origins and delve into its essential components that have garnered acclaim from nutritionists and health enthusiasts alike.

A Historical Voyage

The **Mediterranean diet** is rooted in the traditional culinary patterns of the countries bordering the Mediterranean Sea, including Greece, Italy, and Spain. Historically, this diet evolved from the necessity of local resources, influenced by both the unique geography and the climatic conditions of the region.

The ancient Greeks revered the concept of a balanced diet and believed in the synergistic relationship between food, physical activity, and mental well-being. The Romans later adopted and expanded upon these dietary principles, infusing their culinary culture. As time progressed, various civilizations that traded with or invaded the Mediterranean region introduced new foods and culinary techniques, further enriching the diet.

The Pillars of the Mediterranean Diet

The Mediterranean diet is characterized by a plethora of fresh, nutrient-rich, and flavorful ingredients. Here are the primary components that form its foundation:

1. **Vegetables and Fruits**: These are the cornerstone of the Mediterranean diet. Consumed in abundance, they provide essential vitamins, minerals, and fiber. The focus is on seasonal and locally-sourced produce, ensuring maximum freshness and nutrient retention.

2. **Whole Grains:** Unlike refined grains, whole grains like barley, bulgur, and farro retain their nutrient-rich germ, bran, and endosperm. They provide sustained energy and are rich in fiber, which aids digestion and promotes heart health.

3. **Healthy Fats:** Olive oil, a staple in Mediterranean cuisine, is a primary source of fat. Rich in monounsaturated fats and antioxidants, it's associated with reduced risk of chronic diseases. Nuts and seeds, like almonds and flaxseeds, also provide healthy fats and protein.

4. **Fish and Seafood:** With the Mediterranean Sea at their doorstep, it's no surprise that its inhabitants consume a variety of fish and seafood. These are rich sources of omega-3 fatty acids, known for their heart-protective properties.

5. **Legumes and Pulses:** Beans, lentils, and chickpeas are integral components, offering protein, fiber, and essential minerals. They are often used in soups, stews, and salads.

6. **Dairy:** Fermented dairy products, like yogurt and cheese (especially feta and ricotta), are consumed in moderation. They provide calcium, protein, and probiotics that support gut health.

7. **Herbs and Spices:** Beyond just flavoring dishes, herbs and spices like basil, oregano, rosemary, and saffron have antioxidant properties and potential health benefits.

8. **Wine:** Consumed in moderation and often enjoyed with meals, wine, especially red, is rich in antioxidants like resveratrol, which might offer cardiovascular benefits.

9. **Minimal Red Meat:** Red meat is consumed infrequently and in small portions. The emphasis is on lean cuts, with poultry being preferred over red meats.

10. **Sweets:** Desserts in the Mediterranean diet, such as baklava or figs drizzled with honey, are often fruit-based and use natural sweeteners. They're savored occasionally rather than daily.

The Essence Beyond Ingredients

The Mediterranean diet transcends beyond just the foods consumed. It embodies a way of life that emphasizes the joy of communal eating, savoring each bite, and balancing it with physical activity. The importance of sharing meals with family and friends, coupled with an active lifestyle, is as integral to this diet as the foods themselves.

In summary, the Mediterranean diet is a harmonious blend of rich history, flavorful ingredients, and a holistic approach to well-being. As we delve deeper into its benefits in subsequent sections, its status as one of the world's healthiest diets will become even more evident.

Scientific studies on the Mediterranean diet and lifespan

The Mediterranean diet has often been linked with a multitude of health benefits, ranging from improved heart health to cognitive preservation. Its potential influence on longevity, however, is of significant intrigue. Over the years, a series of scientific studies have aimed to unravel this connection. Let's explore some of the most pivotal research that sheds light on the Mediterranean diet's role in promoting a longer and healthier life.

PREDIMED Study: A Landmark Trial

The **PREDIMED** (Prevención con Dieta Mediterránea) trial is arguably one of the most renowned studies on the Mediterranean diet. Spanning almost five years, this study involved over 7,000 participants from Spain. The participants, primarily at risk for cardiovascular disease, were assigned to one of three diets: a Mediterranean diet supplemented with extra virgin olive oil, a Mediterranean diet supplemented with mixed nuts, or a control diet that advised reduced dietary fat.

Findings:

- Both Mediterranean diet groups witnessed a substantial reduction in the risk of major cardiovascular events compared to the control group.
- Further analysis also indicated a lower risk of mortality in the

Mediterranean diet groups, suggesting potential lifespan-enhancing effects.

The HALE Project: Analyzing European Seniors

The **HALE** (Healthy Ageing: a Longitudinal study in Europe) project analyzed individuals aged 70 to 90 from 11 European countries. Researchers aimed to determine the influence of diet, along with other lifestyle factors, on mortality.

Findings:

- Adherence to a Mediterranean diet, along with factors like physical activity and moderate alcohol consumption, was inversely associated with mortality.
- Notably, those who adhered most closely to the Mediterranean diet had a 20% reduced risk of death.

Greek EPIC Cohort: A Broad Perspective

The **Greek segment** of the European Prospective Investigation into Cancer and Nutrition (EPIC) study provided valuable insights. This cohort study involved tracking around 22,000 participants for over a decade.

Findings:

- A one-point increase in the Mediterranean diet score (a system to assess adherence) was associated with a 12% reduction in overall mortality.
- A two-point increase correlated with a significant decrease in both cancer-related and coronary heart disease-related mortality.

Neurological Health and the Mediterranean Diet

While longevity studies offer a glimpse into the diet's lifespan-extending potential, its role in preserving cognitive function is also noteworthy. A study in the **Annals of Neurology** found that individuals adhering closely to the Mediterranean diet had a reduced risk of developing Alzheimer's disease.

Findings:

- Adherents to the diet had a 40% lower risk of Alzheimer's compared to those who did not follow the diet closely.
- The protective effects were particularly pronounced for those who consumed higher amounts of fish, vegetables, and legumes, and lower amounts of dairy and meat.

Concluding Remarks

While numerous factors influence longevity, from genetics to environmental factors, the Mediterranean diet's potential role is undeniable. Scientific studies consistently highlight its benefits in reducing cardiovascular risk, overall mortality, and even preserving cognitive health.

However, it's crucial to note that the Mediterranean diet's true essence lies in its holistic approach. It's not just about individual components, like olive oil or nuts, but a harmonious blend of nutrient-rich foods, lifestyle practices, and the joys of communal dining.

As more research unfolds, the world continues to appreciate the Mediterranean lifestyle's profound ability to enhance the quality and possibly the quantity of life.

Benefits and Potential Drawbacks

The Mediterranean diet, with its rich tapestry of flavors and nutrient-dense components, has been celebrated by nutritionists, health professionals, and the public alike. Numerous studies have highlighted its potential benefits, but like any diet, it's essential to understand its comprehensive impact, both positive and negative. Let's delve into the recognized benefits and explore some potential drawbacks of this renowned diet.

Recognized Benefits

1. **Heart Health:** Perhaps the most acclaimed benefit, the Mediterranean diet is known for its heart-protective properties. High in monounsaturated fats (from olive oil) and omega-3 fatty acids (from fish), it has been linked to reduced levels of LDL (bad cho-

lesterol) and a decreased risk of atherosclerosis and other cardio-vascular diseases.

2. **Weight Management**: The diet's emphasis on whole foods, fiber-rich grains, and legumes can lead to prolonged satiety. Research indicates that people who follow the Mediterranean diet tend to have a reduced risk of developing obesity and metabolic syndrome.

3. **Blood Sugar Regulation**: The Mediterranean diet may offer benefits for blood sugar control and can reduce the risk of type 2 diabetes. Its focus on complex carbohydrates and healthy fats helps stabilize blood sugar levels, reducing insulin resistance.

4. **Cognitive Health**: As previously discussed, there's promising evidence that the diet can protect against cognitive decline. The antioxidants and anti-inflammatory compounds found in many of its staples, such as olive oil, nuts, and fish, may offer a protective shield for the brain.

5. **Reduced Cancer Risk**: The diet's richness in antioxidants, vitamins, and minerals can lower the risk of certain cancers. Components like lycopene from tomatoes and polyphenols from olive oil have shown potential anticancer properties.

6. **Digestive Health**: The abundance of fiber from fruits, vegetables, and whole grains aids digestion and promotes a healthy gut. This can lead to reduced risks of gastrointestinal conditions like diverticulitis.

Potential Drawbacks

1. **Caloric Density**: While the diet is nutrient-dense, some components, like olive oil and nuts, are also calorie-dense. Without mindful consumption, it might lead to inadvertent calorie over-consumption.

2. **Cost**: Fresh fish, quality olive oils, and organic produce can be expensive. Depending on the region, adhering strictly to the Mediterranean diet might strain some budgets.

3. **Potential for Nutrient Imbalance**: If not varied, any diet can lead to certain nutrient deficiencies. For instance, limited consumption of red meat might lead to lower levels of certain nutrients like iron, vitamin B12, and zinc.

4. **Cultural Adaptation**: The Mediterranean diet reflects the culinary habits of specific regions. People from different cultural backgrounds might find it challenging to adapt wholly, potentially missing out on some benefits.

5. **Wine Misinterpretation**: While moderate wine consumption is a part of the diet, excessive or inappropriate consumption can negate the benefits and introduce health risks, especially for those with a predisposition to alcohol addiction.

Striking a Balance

Like any dietary approach, the key with the Mediterranean diet is balance and adaptability. While the benefits are significant and backed by extensive research, it's crucial for individuals to adapt it according to their needs, preferences, and local availability of ingredients.

In conclusion, the Mediterranean diet stands out as a shining example of a dietary pattern that can enhance health and potentially extend life. Recognizing its few drawbacks and addressing them mindfully can allow individuals to harvest its myriad benefits while maintaining a balanced and joyous relationship with food.

Chapter 3:
Vegan and Vegetarian Diets

Origins and key differences between veganism and vegetarianism

As societies grapple with the challenges of sustainable living, ethical consumption, and health, veganism and vegetarianism have gained significant traction. These diets are no longer seen as mere trends but as established dietary patterns with deep-rooted histories. To appreciate their nuances and impacts, we must first understand their origins and the distinctions between them.

Origins of Vegetarianism

Vegetarianism, in its broadest sense, is the practice of abstaining from consuming meat. Its origins are ancient and intertwined with religious, philosophical, and health considerations.

1. **Religious Roots:** Many ancient religions, including Hinduism, Buddhism, and Jainism, have advocated for a vegetarian diet based on the principles of non-violence (ahimsa) and reverence for all living beings. The abstinence from meat, especially in Brahminical traditions in India, dates back thousands of years.

2. **Philosophical Stances:** In ancient Greece, notable figures like Pythagoras and Plato promoted vegetarianism. Their motivations ranged from the belief in the transmigration of souls to the conviction that a vegetarian diet supported a balanced mind and body.

3. **Modern Movements:** The 19th and 20th centuries witnessed a resurgence of vegetarianism in the West. Associations like the Vegetarian Society in England, established in the mid-1800s, promoted the diet for health, ethical, and environmental reasons.

Origins of Veganism

Veganism is a more recent offshoot of vegetarianism. While vegetarians might consume dairy products, eggs, or both, vegans abstain from all animal-derived products.

1. **Ethical Beginnings**: The term "vegan" was coined in 1944 by Donald Watson, a member of the Vegetarian Society. Disheartened by the ethical implications of dairy and egg production, Watson and like-minded vegetarians established The Vegan Society. Their motivations extended beyond diet, encompassing a broader lifestyle choice against all forms of animal exploitation.

2. **Modern Awareness**: With increasing exposure to industrial farming practices and their implications on animal welfare, the environment, and health, veganism has seen exponential growth in the 21st century.

Key Differences Between Veganism and Vegetarianism

1. **Dietary Restrictions:**

- **Vegetarians** exclude meat, poultry, and fish from their diet. However, there are variations within vegetarianism:

- **Lacto-Vegetarians** consume dairy but avoid eggs.

- **Ovo-Vegetarians** eat eggs but not dairy.

- **Lacto-Ovo Vegetarians** include both dairy and eggs in their diet.

- **Vegans** avoid all animal-derived products, including meat, dairy, eggs, and often honey.

2. **Motivations:**

- **Vegetarians** primarily abstain from meat for health, religious, or ethical reasons.

- **Vegans** often extend their motivations beyond diet, embracing a lifestyle that opposes all forms of animal exploitation, including clothing (like leather and wool) and entertainment (such as circuses or zoos).

3. **Nutritional Considerations:**

- **Vegetarians** can obtain certain nutrients like vitamin B12, calcium, and omega-3 fatty acids from dairy or eggs.

- **Vegans** need to be more vigilant about their nutrient sources, often requiring fortified foods or supplements to ensure they meet all their dietary needs.

4. **Environmental Impact:**

- Both diets, when compared to a typical omnivorous diet, have a lower environmental footprint in terms of water usage, greenhouse gas emissions, and land use. However, veganism, by eschewing all animal-derived products, often has an even lower impact.

In conclusion, while veganism and vegetarianism share a common thread of minimizing or eliminating meat consumption, they have distinct origins, motivations, and dietary implications. Recognizing these nuances is crucial for anyone considering adopting or studying these dietary patterns.

Studies relating vegan/vegetarian diets to longevity

The vegan and vegetarian diets have gained prominence not just for ethical and environmental reasons, but also for their potential health benefits. A key question many researchers have sought to address is whether these plant-based diets can enhance longevity. Let's delve into some of the pivotal studies that have explored this connection.

The Adventist Health Studies

One of the most comprehensive studies on vegetarianism and longevity comes from the Seventh-day Adventists, a religious group that often promotes vegetarianism. The **Adventist Health Studies**, which began in the 1970s, have involved tens of thousands of participants and spanned several decades.

Findings:

- Vegetarians in the study had a 12% lower risk of mortality compared to non-vegetarians.
- The benefits were more pronounced for specific causes of death, such as heart disease and kidney-related complications.
- Vegan participants had lower rates of total cancer compared to non-vegetarians.

The European Prospective Investigation into Cancer and Nutrition (EPIC-Oxford)

Another large-scale study, the **EPIC-Oxford**, tracked the dietary patterns and health outcomes of thousands of participants in the UK.

Findings:

- Vegetarians had a 32% lower risk of hospitalization or death from heart disease than meat-eaters.
- Both vegans and vegetarians had lower cholesterol and blood pressure levels, reducing cardiovascular disease risks.
- However, there were no significant differences in overall mortality between the diet groups.

The Blue Zones Study

The **Blue Zones** are regions identified worldwide where people live significantly longer than average. While not all inhabitants of these zones are strictly vegetarian, their diets are predominantly plant-based.

Findings:

- The diets of Blue Zone residents are rich in legumes, whole grains, vegetables, and fruits, with minimal animal products.

- Factors like strong social connections, physical activity, and a sense of purpose also play a role in their longevity, but diet is considered a key contributor.

Potential Concerns and Counter Studies

While many studies highlight the benefits of vegan and vegetarian diets, some also raise concerns.

1. **Bone Health**: A segment of the EPIC-Oxford study found that vegans had a 30% higher risk of bone fractures than meat-eaters, likely due to lower calcium intake.

2. **Nutrient Deficiency**: There are concerns that strict vegan diets might lead to deficiencies in nutrients like vitamin B12, iron, omega-3 fatty acids, and protein. However, well-planned vegan diets can address these potential gaps.

3. **Generalizability**: It's worth noting that many of the health benefits observed in vegetarians and vegans could be influenced by their overall healthier lifestyle choices, such as reduced smoking, regular exercise, and limited alcohol consumption.

Concluding Remarks

On balance, vegan and vegetarian diets, when well-planned and combined with other healthy lifestyle practices, have shown potential in reducing the risk of chronic diseases and potentially enhancing longevity. The antioxidant-rich, low-saturated fat, and high-fiber nature of these diets play a role in these observed benefits.

However, individual nutritional needs and health considerations should be factored in. It's also essential to remember that while diet plays a significant role in health and longevity, other factors, from genetics to socio-economic conditions, also come into play.

For anyone considering these diets, consulting with a nutrition professional can ensure a balanced and healthful approach that maximizes the potential benefits while addressing any concerns.

Nutritional considerations for those adopting these diets

Embracing a vegan or vegetarian diet can lead to various health benefits, as highlighted by numerous studies. However, ensuring that the diet is nutritionally complete is crucial to harnessing these benefits while avoiding potential pitfalls. This section will discuss the essential nutritional considerations for those transitioning to or maintaining a vegan or vegetarian lifestyle.

1. Protein

Vegetarians: Can obtain protein from dairy products, eggs, legumes, nuts, seeds, and whole grains.

Vegans: Need to be more conscious of protein sources, focusing on legumes (like lentils, chickpeas, and black beans), tofu, tempeh, quinoa, hemp seeds, and seitan.

Tip: A combination of different plant-based proteins throughout the day ensures a balance of essential amino acids.

2. Iron

Plant-based diets offer iron in the non-heme form, which is less efficiently absorbed than the heme iron found in meat.

Sources: Lentils, chickpeas, tofu, quinoa, chia seeds, hemp seeds, spinach, and fortified cereals.

Tip: Consuming iron-rich foods with vitamin C (like citrus fruits or bell peppers) can enhance iron absorption. It's also wise to avoid drinking tea or coffee with iron-rich meals as they can inhibit absorption.

3. Vitamin B12

This vitamin is primarily found in animal products, so supplementation is often recommended for vegans and sometimes for vegetarians.

Vegetarians: Can obtain B12 from dairy products and eggs.

Vegans: Should consider fortified foods (like plant-based milk or cereals) or a B12 supplement.

Tip: Regularly monitor B12 levels, especially for those on a strict vegan diet.

4. Omega-3 Fatty Acids

While fish is a primary source of omega-3s, plant-based alternatives exist.

Sources: Flaxseeds, chia seeds, hemp seeds, walnuts, and algae-based supplements.

Tip: Algal oil supplements can provide the essential EPA and DHA forms of omega-3s, which are often missing in vegan diets.

5. Calcium

Though dairy is a well-known calcium source, several plant-based alternatives are available.

Sources: Tofu, fortified plant milks, almonds, tahini, collard greens, turnip greens, chia seeds, and figs.

Tip: For those avoiding dairy, it's beneficial to include multiple calcium sources in the daily diet and consider fortified foods or supplements if needed.

6. Vitamin D

Often dubbed the "sunshine vitamin," it plays a role in calcium absorption and overall bone health.

Sources: While sunlight is the primary source, fortified plant-based milk, mushrooms exposed to sunlight, and supplements can help, especially in regions with limited sun exposure.

Tip: Ensure adequate sun exposure, but consider supplements, especially during winter months.

7. Zinc

This mineral is crucial for immune function, metabolic health, and wound healing.

Sources: Whole grains, legumes, nuts, and seeds.

Tip: Similar to iron, the phytates in plant foods can reduce zinc absorption. Soaking, sprouting, or fermenting foods can improve bio-availability.

8. Iodine

Essential for thyroid function, its primary source is seafood. However, alternatives exist.

Sources: Iodized salt, seaweed, and some fortified foods.

Tip: Regularly include small amounts of seaweed, like nori or kelp, in the diet. But be cautious about excessive consumption, which can lead to too much iodine.

Concluding Thoughts

Transitioning to a vegan or vegetarian diet requires attention to detail, especially concerning nutrient intake. However, with proper planning, knowledge, and possibly some supplementation, these diets can be both nutritionally complete and health-promoting. It's always advisable for individuals to consult with a nutritionist or dietitian, ensuring that they are meeting all their dietary needs.

Chapter 4: Paleo Diet

Origins and key components

The Paleo Diet, often termed the "Caveman Diet," seeks to emulate the dietary patterns of our pre-agricultural, hunter-gatherer ancestors. Its proponents argue that this way of eating is more in line with our genetics, aiming to enhance health by looking to a time before modern diseases became prevalent.

Origins of the Paleo Diet

The foundational premise of the Paleo Diet is rooted in evolutionary biology. It is based on the notion that for the vast majority of human history, agriculture did not exist, and thus humans consumed a diet free from grains, dairy, legumes, and processed foods. It wasn't until the advent of agriculture, around 10,000 years ago, that these food groups became staples in the human diet.

1. **Evolutionary Mismatch Hypothesis:** This concept suggests that many modern diseases stem from a misalignment between our current diet and lifestyle and those of our Paleolithic ancestors. Diseases like obesity, diabetes, and cardiovascular issues, according to proponents, arise from this mismatch.

2. **Modern Emergence:** While the underpinning ideas have been around for a while, the Paleo Diet's popularity surged in the late 20th and early 21st centuries. Dr. Loren Cordain's book, "The Paleo Diet," published in 2002, is credited with popularizing this dietary approach.

Key Components of the Paleo Diet

To align with what is believed to have been the Paleolithic human's diet, the Paleo Diet emphasizes whole foods while eliminating certain food groups. Here's a breakdown:

3. Foods to Eat:

- **Proteins:** Lean meats, especially grass-fed or wild-caught varieties, are encouraged. This includes beef, lamb, chicken, turkey, pork, and game meats. Fish, particularly those rich in omega-3 fatty acids like salmon, mackerel, and trout, are also recommended.

- **Fruits and Vegetables:** Most fruits and vegetables are considered Paleo-friendly. These provide essential vitamins, minerals, and fiber.

- **Nuts and Seeds:** Almonds, macadamias, walnuts, hazelnuts, sunflower seeds, and pumpkin seeds are popular choices. However, they should be consumed in moderation due to their high-calorie content.

- **Healthy Fats:** Olive oil, coconut oil, avocado oil, and flaxseed oil are favored, emphasizing the importance of omega-3 to omega-6 fatty acid balance.

- **Eggs:** Especially those from free-range or pasture-raised chickens.

4. Foods to Avoid:

- **Grains:** This includes wheat, rice, barley, oats, and any products made from these, like bread and pasta.

- **Legumes:** Beans, lentils, peanuts, and soy products are excluded.

- **Dairy:** Most Paleo diets avoid dairy, especially from processed and pasteurized sources. However, some versions allow full-fat and fermented dairy products.

- **Refined Sugars and Artificial Sweeteners:** Honey and maple syrup might be used sparingly, but refined sugars, high fructose corn syrup, and artificial sweeteners are out.

- **Processed Foods:** Anything with additives, preservatives, or artificial ingredients doesn't fit the Paleo profile.

- **Trans Fats and Vegetable Oils:** These include margarine, hydrogenated oils, and oils high in omega-6, like soybean and corn oil.

5. **Alcohol and Caffeine:** While our ancestors likely didn't consume these, some modern interpretations of the Paleo diet allow beverages like red wine (in moderation) and green tea, emphasizing their potential health benefits.

Concluding Thoughts

The Paleo Diet harks back to an imagined pre-agricultural era, emphasizing foods that could be hunted or gathered. Its emphasis on whole foods and the avoidance of processed items aligns it with many principles of healthy eating. However, as with all diets, individual adaptations and consultation with nutrition experts can ensure it's followed in a balanced and healthful manner.

Analysis of research on the Paleo diet's impact on lifespan

The Paleo Diet has gained significant attention for its potential health benefits. As with any dietary approach, understanding its scientific basis is crucial, especially when considering long-term impacts such as lifespan. Here, we dive into research findings regarding the Paleo Diet's implications for longevity.

Cardiovascular Health

A predominant area of interest is how the Paleo Diet affects cardiovascular health, a significant determinant of lifespan.

- **Positive Findings:** Some studies suggest that the Paleo Diet can reduce risk factors for cardiovascular disease. Lindeberg et al. (2007) found that a Paleolithic diet improved glucose tolerance and reduced waist circumference, blood pressure, and levels of plasminogen activator inhibitor-1 (a marker of heart disease risk) compared to a Mediterranean-like diet.

- **Areas of Caution:** The emphasis on red meat in some interpretations of the Paleo Diet could be of concern, as excessive consumption has been linked to heart disease in various studies. However, it's important to note that the Paleo Diet encourages lean, grass-fed, or wild-caught meats, which have a different nutritional profile than conventionally raised meats.

Metabolic Health and Obesity

Obesity and metabolic syndrome are significant factors influencing lifespan and quality of life.

- **Positive Findings**: A study by Frassetto et al. (2009) discovered that participants on a Paleolithic diet for ten days showed improved blood pressure, insulin sensitivity, and lipid profiles, all of which are crucial markers for metabolic health.

- **Areas of Caution**: While short-term interventions have shown benefits, long-term studies on the Paleo Diet's impact on metabolic health and weight maintenance are still sparse. Sustainability is key to any diet's success in this arena.

Bone Health

Given that dairy, a primary calcium source for many, is excluded in the Paleo Diet, concerns arise about bone health.

- **Positive Findings**: The diet's emphasis on vegetables, nuts, and seeds can provide calcium. Additionally, the reduction in sodium and increase in potassium can support better calcium retention and bone health.

- **Areas of Caution**: Despite these potential benefits, adequate calcium intake remains a concern, especially over the long term. Monitoring and possibly supplementing might be necessary.

Longevity Markers

Examining factors directly linked to longevity provides insights into a diet's potential lifespan impact.

- **Positive Findings**: A study by Osterdahl et al. (2008) over a three-week period found that a Paleolithic diet reduced blood pressure, total cholesterol, and LDL levels, while increasing levels of protective antioxidants and clot-dissolving substances. Such markers are often associated with longevity.

- **Areas of Caution**: The diet's long-term impact on these markers remains uncertain. Additionally, potential increases in meat consumption could elevate levels of IGF-1, a growth hormone linked to certain cancers, although the relevance of this in the context of the Paleo Diet requires more investigation.

Concluding Thoughts

The current body of research offers mixed insights into the Paleo Diet's impact on lifespan. While certain markers of health and longevity seem to benefit from this dietary approach, long-term studies are needed. As with any diet, individual variations and holistic considerations (such as exercise, stress management, and sleep) play pivotal roles in determining overall health and longevity outcomes. For those considering the Paleo Diet, it's always recommended to consult with healthcare professionals to tailor the approach to individual needs and ensure balanced nutrition.

Strengths and weaknesses of the Paleo approach

The Paleo Diet, like any dietary approach, has its advocates and detractors. To make an informed decision about adopting this diet, it's important to understand its strengths and weaknesses. This balanced perspective can guide individuals in tailoring the diet to their unique needs.

Strengths of the Paleo Diet

1. **Emphasis on Whole Foods**: At its core, the Paleo Diet promotes the consumption of unprocessed, nutrient-dense foods. This emphasis on whole foods naturally reduces intake of additives, preservatives, and unhealthy trans fats often found in processed foods.

2. **Potential for Weight Loss**: Several studies have demonstrated weight loss and improved body composition among participants following the Paleo Diet, especially when compared to standard Western diets. The focus on protein and healthy fats can increase satiety, potentially reducing overall caloric intake.

3. **Improved Metabolic Health**: As previously discussed, some research indicates that the Paleo Diet can lead to improvements in metabolic markers such as insulin sensitivity, blood pressure, and lipid profiles.

4. **Reduction in Inflammatory Foods**: By eliminating grains and legumes, which contain anti-nutrients like lectins and phytates, the Paleo Diet may reduce sources of inflammation for some people. This can be especially beneficial for those with autoimmune or inflammatory conditions.

5. **Flexibility**: While there are foundational principles, there's flexibility in the Paleo approach, allowing individuals to tailor the diet based on personal preferences and tolerances.

Weaknesses of the Paleo Diet

1. **Potential Nutrient Deficiencies**: The exclusion of certain food groups, such as dairy and grains, can lead to potential deficiencies in calcium and certain B vitamins. While these nutrients can be sourced from alternative foods, it requires careful planning.

2. **High Meat Consumption Concerns**: While advocates stress the importance of lean and grass-fed meats, excessive consumption of red meat is still a concern for some health professionals due to potential associations with heart disease and certain cancers.

3. **Sustainability and Practicality**: For many, adhering to the strict guidelines of the Paleo Diet can be challenging over the long term, especially in social settings or when dining out. Additionally, sourcing grass-fed meats or organic produce consistently can be costly.

4. **Lack of Long-term Research**: While short-term studies have shown benefits, there's a lack of comprehensive long-term research on the Paleo Diet's impact on lifespan and chronic disease prevention.

5. **Evolutionary Assumptions**: Critics argue that the diet is based on certain assumptions about Paleolithic-era eating habits that

might not be entirely accurate. For instance, early humans' diets varied greatly depending on their geographic location and availability of resources.

Concluding Thoughts

The Paleo Diet's strengths lie in its promotion of whole foods, potential metabolic benefits, and adaptability. However, potential nutrient deficiencies, concerns over high meat consumption, and questions about its long-term sustainability and evolutionary basis present challenges. As with any dietary approach, individuals should weigh these strengths and weaknesses against their personal health goals, needs, and lifestyle. Consulting with a nutritionist or healthcare professional can provide further guidance and ensure a balanced approach to the Paleo Diet.

Chapter 5:
Ketogenic Diet

What is ketosis? How does it impact the body?

The Ketogenic Diet, commonly referred to as the "Keto Diet", revolves around the concept of ketosis. This metabolic state has been the subject of much intrigue and research, especially given its potential health implications. But what exactly is ketosis, and how does it influence the body?

Understanding Ketosis

Ketosis is a metabolic state in which the body primarily uses ketone bodies – compounds produced in the liver from fatty acids – for energy, rather than relying on glucose from carbohydrates. This shift occurs when carbohydrate intake is significantly reduced.

   Mechanism:

1. **Carbohydrate Restriction:** When dietary carbohydrates are limited, the body's glucose reserves begin to deplete. This depletion results in a decrease in insulin levels, prompting the body to start breaking down stored fat into molecules called fatty acids and glycerol.

2. **Ketone Production:** The liver converts some of these fatty acids into three primary types of ketone bodies: acetone, acetoacetate, and beta-hydroxybutyrate. These ketones then serve as an alternative fuel source for various tissues, especially the brain.

How Ketosis Impacts the Body

1. **Brain Function:** The brain is a glucose-dependent organ, but it can derive up to 70% of its energy from ketones when glucose supplies are limited. This shift can lead to improved mental clarity and focus for some people. It's also being explored as a therapeu-

tic strategy for neurological disorders like epilepsy, Alzheimer's disease, and Parkinson's disease.

2. **Weight Loss:** One of the primary reasons many adopt a ketogenic diet is for weight loss. By using stored fat as energy, body fat percentage can decrease. Moreover, ketosis often suppresses appetite, possibly due to changes in hunger hormones, making calorie restriction easier.

3. **Blood Sugar and Insulin Regulation:** The ketogenic diet can lead to reduced blood sugar and insulin levels, potentially benefiting those with type 2 diabetes or at risk of the disease.

4. **Enhanced Energy:** Some individuals report sustained energy levels while in ketosis, as the body has a steady fuel supply from ketones, and there aren't the typical blood sugar spikes and dips associated with a high-carb diet.

5. **Improved Lipid Profiles:** There's evidence to suggest that the ketogenic diet can increase levels of high-density lipoprotein (HDL, or "good" cholesterol) and decrease levels of low-density lipoprotein (LDL, or "bad" cholesterol), potentially reducing the risk of cardiovascular diseases.

6. **Inflammation Reduction:** Research suggests that ketosis may reduce systemic inflammation, a key contributor to chronic diseases. This might be due to a decrease in the production of reactive oxygen species and an increase in the production of antioxidants.

7. **Muscle Preservation:** While weight loss diets often lead to muscle loss alongside fat loss, the ketogenic diet's emphasis on protein and its muscle-sparing properties can help preserve muscle mass.

Points of Caution

While ketosis has its benefits, it's essential to be aware of potential side effects. Some people experience the "keto flu" as their body adjusts, which can include symptoms like headache, fatigue, nausea, dizziness, and irritability. Proper hydration and electrolyte balance can mitigate these effects. Additionally, the long-term impacts of a ketogenic diet on health are still under research, and it's vital to approach the diet with informed guidance.

Concluding Thoughts

Ketosis is a powerful metabolic state with wide-ranging effects on the body. While it offers several benefits, especially for brain function, weight loss, and metabolic health, individual responses can vary. Those interested in a ketogenic diet should seek guidance to ensure they're achieving ketosis safely and effectively.

Research on the Keto diet's relation to lifespan

The Ketogenic Diet has been lauded for its potential health benefits, particularly in metabolic and neurological contexts. Yet, an intriguing area of exploration is its potential impact on lifespan and longevity. The association between the Keto diet and longevity emerges from a blend of direct research and extrapolations from related studies.

Caloric Restriction and Lifespan

Historically, caloric restriction (CR) without malnutrition has been the most consistent dietary intervention associated with increased lifespan in various organisms. The mechanisms believed to be responsible include reduced oxidative stress, enhanced autophagy, and improved mitochondrial function.

The Keto diet can mimic some of the metabolic effects of caloric restriction. For instance, both CR and the Keto diet increase levels of the ketone body beta-hydroxybutyrate (BHB), which has various beneficial effects, such as reducing inflammation and oxidative stress.

Direct Research on Keto and Lifespan

- **Animal Studies**: A 2017 study published in the journal *Cell Metabolism* found that mice fed a ketogenic diet lived longer and had better motor function and cognitive health than mice on a standard diet. While the mice on the Keto diet didn't eat fewer calories, they still experienced some benefits typically associated with caloric restriction.

- **Human Data**: Long-term studies on the ketogenic diet's effects on human lifespan directly are currently limited. However, given the positive impacts of the diet on several health markers, there's potential for an indirect association.

Keto's Impact on Age-related Diseases

A strong determinant of lifespan is the onset and progression of age-related diseases. By influencing these, the Keto diet could indirectly affect longevity.

- **Neuroprotective Effects**: The Keto diet's neuroprotective benefits might delay the onset of neurodegenerative diseases like Alzheimer's and Parkinson's. This is likely due to enhanced brain energy metabolism from ketone bodies and reduced neuroinflammation.

- **Cancer**: Some preliminary studies suggest that the Keto diet might slow the progression of certain cancers, given that many cancer cells predominantly metabolize glucose for growth. However, this area requires more research, as the diet's impact might vary depending on the type of cancer.

- **Metabolic Health**: By improving markers of metabolic health, like insulin sensitivity and blood lipid profiles, the Keto diet could potentially reduce the risk of heart disease and type 2 diabetes, prominent factors influencing lifespan.

Potential Downsides and Considerations

It's essential to approach the association between the Keto diet and lifespan with a balanced perspective.

- **Diet Composition**: Not all ketogenic diets are the same. A diet high in saturated fats and low in fibrous vegetables might not offer the same lifespan benefits as a well-formulated ketogenic diet rich in unsaturated fats and nutrient-dense plants.

- **Individual Variability**: The effects of the Keto diet can vary significantly between individuals, influenced by genetics, gut microbiota, and other factors. As such, its impact on lifespan could differ across populations.

Concluding Thoughts

While preliminary research, especially in animal models, suggests potential lifespan-extending effects of the Keto diet, direct evidence in humans is still evolving. The diet's potential to mitigate risk factors for age-related diseases provides an optimistic perspective on its implications for longevity. However, as with any dietary approach, individual needs, tolerances, and the diet's composition play pivotal roles in determining overall health outcomes. Continual research in this exciting area holds promise for further insights into the ketogenic diet and longevity.

Benefits and potential concerns

The Ketogenic Diet has surged in popularity, driven in part by a myriad of reported health benefits. As with any dietary approach, the Keto diet has its advantages and potential drawbacks. A comprehensive understanding of both can guide individuals in making informed decisions.

Benefits of the Ketogenic Diet

1. **Weight Loss:** One of the most celebrated benefits of the Keto diet is its potential for weight loss. The diet's macronutrient distribution can lead to increased satiety, making it easier to reduce calorie intake. Additionally, the shift to fat metabolism can enhance fat burning.

2. **Improved Blood Glucose Control:** The diet can lead to stable blood sugar levels, making it an attractive option for individuals with type 2 diabetes or those at risk.

3. **Enhanced Brain Health:** Ketone bodies, especially beta-hydroxybutyrate (BHB), can serve as an efficient fuel for the brain. This has led to the exploration of the Keto diet as a potential therapeutic tool for neurological disorders, including epilepsy, Alzheimer's disease, and Parkinson's disease.

4. **Heart Health:** Some studies suggest improved lipid profiles with increased HDL ("good") cholesterol and decreased LDL ("bad") cholesterol. This can potentially reduce the risk of cardiovascular diseases.

5. **Appetite Suppression:** Many individuals report decreased hunger while on the Keto diet, which can be attributed to increased ketone production and stabilized blood sugar levels.

6. **Anti-Inflammatory Effects:** The diet may reduce systemic inflammation, potentially mitigating the risk of chronic diseases.

Potential Concerns of the Ketogenic Diet

1. **Nutrient Deficiencies:** Given the restrictions on several food groups, there's potential for deficiencies in essential nutrients, including fiber, vitamins, and minerals. For instance, restricting fruits and certain vegetables can limit the intake of vitamin C and potassium.

2. **Keto Flu:** As the body transitions into ketosis, some people experience flu-like symptoms, including headaches, fatigue, dizziness, and irritability. While these symptoms are generally temporary, they can be off-putting.

3. **Liver and Kidney Concerns:** The increased production of ketones can put additional strain on the liver. Furthermore, the diet's high protein content might be challenging for those with kidney issues.

4. **Bone Health:** Some research suggests a potential risk for decreased bone mineral density over extended periods on the diet.

5. **Increased Cholesterol for Some:** While many experience improved cholesterol profiles, a subset of individuals might see elevated cholesterol levels on a Keto diet, particularly if there's a heavy reliance on saturated fats.

6. **Long-Term Sustainability:** The restrictive nature of the diet can be challenging for some to maintain over the long term. This can lead to yo-yo dieting, which has its own set of health concerns.

7. **Gastrointestinal Issues:** Due to the low fiber intake, some individuals experience constipation or other gastrointestinal disturbances when on the Keto diet.

Concluding Thoughts

The Ketogenic Diet offers a range of potential benefits, especially for weight loss, brain health, and metabolic regulation. However, its restrictive nature presents challenges and potential health concerns. It's imperative for those considering or adopting the Keto diet to approach it with a well-informed perspective, incorporating a variety of nutrient-dense foods and, if necessary, supplements to ensure a balanced nutrient intake. Consulting with healthcare professionals can offer personalized guidance, ensuring the diet's benefits are maximized while minimizing potential risks.

Chapter 6:
Plant-based Whole Foods Diet

Definition and core principles

The Plant-based Whole Foods Diet (PBWF) emphasizes the consumption of natural, unprocessed foods primarily derived from plants. As concerns grow regarding the health implications of processed foods and certain animal products, the PBWF diet has garnered significant attention. Let's delve into its definition and core principles to understand its essence.

Definition of the Plant-based Whole Foods Diet

The Plant-based Whole Foods Diet is characterized by its focus on consuming foods in their most natural state, avoiding processed foods and animal-derived products. It is a holistic approach that goes beyond just eating plants; it emphasizes the quality, source, and preparation of the food.

Core Principles

1. **Emphasis on Whole Foods**: The diet prioritizes foods that are unrefined or minimally refined. This means opting for brown rice over white rice, whole fruits instead of fruit juices, and consuming whole grains, legumes, nuts, and seeds in their most natural forms.

2. **Predominantly Plant-based**: While the diet does not necessarily exclude all animal products, it encourages a primary focus on plant-derived foods. This encompasses vegetables, fruits, whole grains, nuts, seeds, and legumes.

3. **Minimizing Processed Foods**: Highly processed foods, even those that are plant-based, are typically reduced or eliminated in this diet. This includes foods like refined sugars, processed oils, and artificial additives.

4. **No Refined Sugars**: Sugars in the PBWF diet come from whole food sources, like fruits and certain grains. Refined sugars, including high fructose corn syrup and white table sugar, are excluded due to their association with various health issues.

5. **Natural Fats**: Instead of processed oils and fats, the diet emphasizes obtaining fats from whole food sources such as avocados, nuts, and seeds.

6. **Hydration from Natural Sources**: Instead of sugary drinks or sodas, hydration is emphasized through water, herbal teas, and natural beverages like unsweetened coconut water.

7. **Limiting Salt Intake**: While some salt is essential for bodily functions, excessive salt consumption is discouraged. Instead, flavoring foods with herbs, spices, and natural seasonings is promoted.

8. **Mindful Consumption**: The PBWF diet often integrates principles of mindful eating, encouraging individuals to be present during meals, savoring each bite, and listening to their bodies' hunger and fullness cues.

9. **Sustainable and Ethical Choices**: Many proponents of the PBWF diet emphasize not only personal health but also the health of the planet. This translates to choosing sustainably sourced produce, reducing plastic and waste, and considering the ethical implications of food choices.

Concluding Thoughts

The Plant-based Whole Foods Diet offers a comprehensive approach to nutrition and well-being. It goes beyond mere food selection, intertwining principles of health, sustainability, and mindfulness. By focusing on unprocessed, plant-derived foods, the diet encourages consumption patterns associated with numerous health benefits, from weight management to chronic disease prevention.

Incorporating the principles of the PBWF diet does not demand perfection or complete exclusion of all processed or animal-derived foods for everyone. Instead, it provides a guiding framework, allowing individuals to make informed choices that align with their health goals and ethical beliefs.

Exploration of studies on lifespan and this diet

The Plant-based Whole Foods Diet (PBWF) has become a focal point in nutritional research due to its potential health benefits. Specifically, numerous studies have delved into the correlation between this diet and its implications for longevity and healthspan. Here, we will explore the salient findings from research examining the potential lifespan-extending benefits of the PBWF diet.

Epidemiological Evidence

1. **Blue Zones Studies**: Blue Zones refer to regions in the world where an unusually high proportion of people live past the age of 100. Notably, these areas include Sardinia (Italy), Okinawa (Japan), Loma Linda (California, USA), the Nicoya Peninsula (Costa Rica), and Ikaria (Greece). One common dietary pattern observed across these regions is a high consumption of plant-based foods, particularly legumes, whole grains, and vegetables, with minimal processed foods.

2. **Adventist Health Studies**: Loma Linda, California, home to a significant Seventh-day Adventist population, offers invaluable insights into the PBWF diet. These studies have consistently found that vegetarians and vegans within this community have a lower risk of many chronic diseases and live longer than their non-vegetarian counterparts. The emphasis on whole, plant-based foods in their diet is believed to contribute significantly to these health outcomes.

Clinical Trials and Longitudinal Studies

1. **The China Study**: Often referred to as one of the most comprehensive nutritional studies ever undertaken, The China Study investigated the relationship between diet and chronic diseases

in rural China. Findings suggested that regions with a higher consumption of plant-based foods had lower rates of heart disease, cancer, and other chronic conditions.

2. **HEART Trials:** Dr. Dean Ornish's Lifestyle Heart Trials demonstrated that a low-fat, plant-based whole foods diet, combined with other lifestyle changes, could reverse heart disease in certain patients. While not exclusively focused on lifespan, the implication is that by reducing and even reversing heart disease, one of the leading causes of death, the potential for a longer life is increased.

3. **EPIC-Oxford Study:** This European study followed thousands of participants, including vegetarians, vegans, and meat-eaters, to compare health outcomes. Results indicated that those following plant-based diets had lower overall mortality rates, suggesting a link between these dietary patterns and increased lifespan.

Biological Mechanisms

While epidemiological and clinical studies provide observational and interventional insights, understanding the biological mechanisms is essential. Research indicates that plant-based diets:

- Reduce oxidative stress and inflammation, both implicated in aging.
- Enhance telomere length, which is associated with cellular aging.
- Improve gut microbiota diversity, which plays a role in overall health and longevity.

Concluding Thoughts

The accumulated evidence from diverse research methodologies strongly suggests a positive association between the Plant-based Whole Foods Diet and longevity. While causation is challenging to determine in nutritional studies due to numerous confounding factors, the consistent patterns observed across different populations and settings lend significant credence to the potential lifespan-extending benefits of the PBWF diet.

As always, it's important to remember that diet is just one piece of the longevity puzzle, and its effects are likely to be most pronounced when combined with other healthy lifestyle practices, such as regular exercise, stress management, and avoiding harmful habits like smoking or excessive alcohol consumption.

Comparison to vegetarian and vegan diets

The landscape of plant-centric diets is vast and varied. While the Plant-based Whole Foods Diet (PBWF) shares many principles with vegetarianism and veganism, each has its unique characteristics, purposes, and nutritional considerations. This section delves into a comparative analysis of the PBWF diet with its vegetarian and vegan counterparts to discern their similarities and differences.

Similarities

1. **Predominant Focus on Plant-derived Foods**: All three diets center around foods derived from plants, including fruits, vegetables, legumes, grains, nuts, and seeds.

2. **Potential Health Benefits**: Research indicates that people following any of these diets tend to have a lower risk of many chronic diseases, including heart disease, hypertension, certain cancers, and type 2 diabetes.

3. **Environmental and Ethical Considerations**: Many proponents of these diets emphasize the environmental advantages of reduced meat consumption and the ethical aspects concerning animal welfare.

Differences

1. **Animal Products:**

- **PBWF**: While the PBWF diet primarily focuses on plant-derived foods, it does not inherently exclude all animal products. However, it emphasizes their minimal consumption and, when included, stresses choosing ethically-sourced, free-range, or organic options.

- **Vegetarian:** Vegetarians abstain from consuming meat, poultry, and fish. However, they may consume dairy products and eggs.

- **Vegan:** Vegans avoid all animal-derived products, including dairy, eggs, and honey. Their diet is exclusively plant-based.

2. Processed Foods:

- **PBWF:** A distinctive feature of the PBWF diet is its staunch opposition to processed foods, even if they're plant-based. This means items like processed vegan cheeses, mock meats, and refined sugars are typically excluded.

- **Vegetarian/Vegan:** While many vegetarians and vegans prioritize whole foods, these diets do not inherently exclude processed or refined foods, provided they don't contain animal-derived ingredients.

3. Nutritional Emphasis:

- **PBWF:** This diet emphasizes nutrient density and holistic health. It promotes consuming a variety of whole foods to ensure a comprehensive nutrient intake.

- **Vegetarian/Vegan:** While these diets can be nutrient-dense, they don't always inherently emphasize whole foods. It's possible to be a vegan or vegetarian and consume a diet high in processed foods and sugars.

4. Reasons for Adoption:

- **PBWF:** People typically choose this diet for a combination of health, environmental, and ethical reasons. The focus is often on long-term health outcomes and sustainability.

- **Vegetarian/Vegan:** These diets are adopted for various reasons, ranging from health concerns to strong ethical beliefs about animal rights. Environmental considerations also play a role for many individuals.

Concluding Thoughts

While the Plant-based Whole Foods Diet, vegetarianism, and veganism all advocate for increased plant food consumption, their motivations, and dietary specifics can vary. It's crucial for individuals to determine which approach aligns best with their personal health goals, ethical beliefs, and lifestyle.

For those concerned primarily with health outcomes, the PBWF diet offers a compelling framework, emphasizing the quality and source of food, irrespective of its plant or animal origin. On the other hand, those driven by ethical considerations might naturally gravitate towards veganism.

Ultimately, it's essential to remember that any dietary shift towards more whole, plant-based foods is likely a step in a positive direction for both individual health and planetary well-being.

Chapter 7:
Intermittent Fasting and Caloric Restriction

Differences between intermittent fasting and caloric restriction

Intermittent Fasting (IF) and Caloric Restriction (CR) are two dietary approaches that have gained considerable attention in the world of health and wellness, particularly for their potential longevity-enhancing benefits. Both modalities center on limiting food intake but do so in distinct ways, leading to unique physiological effects and user experiences. This section will highlight the key differences between IF and CR.

Duration and Timing of Food Restriction

1. **Intermittent Fasting (IF):**

- **Nature:** IF involves cycling between periods of eating and fasting.

- **Examples:** Common patterns include the 16/8 method (16 hours of fasting followed by an 8-hour eating window), the 5:2 diet (eat normally for 5 days and severely restrict calories on 2 non-consecutive days), and alternate-day fasting.

- **Key Aspect:** The emphasis is on *when* you eat, not necessarily *how much* you eat during the eating window.

2. **Caloric Restriction (CR):**

- **Nature:** CR requires consistently reducing daily caloric intake without malnutrition or deprivation of essential nutrients.

- **Typical Reduction:** Often, this is a 20-40% reduction from an individual's typical caloric intake.

- **Key Aspect:** The emphasis is on *how much* you eat daily, irrespective of the eating schedule.

Physiological Responses

1. Intermittent Fasting:

- Initiates processes like autophagy, where cells remove damaged components.

- Can lead to transient metabolic shifts towards fat utilization (ketosis) during prolonged fasting periods.

- May cause more significant short-term fluctuations in blood sugar and insulin levels based on the fasting duration.

2. Caloric Restriction:

- Primarily slows metabolic rate as a response to sustained lower caloric intake.

- Encourages improved cellular efficiency and reduction in oxidative stress.

- Provides a more consistent metabolic environment with less pronounced hormonal fluctuations.

Practical Implications

1. Intermittent Fasting:

- Can be more flexible and easier for some individuals who find it simpler to abstain from eating entirely for specific periods rather than counting calories.

- May lead to overeating during feeding windows if not mindful.

- Might not be suitable for everyone, especially those with certain medical conditions or specific daily routines.

2. Caloric Restriction:

- Requires more consistent tracking and mindfulness about total caloric intake.

- Might be more feasible for those who struggle with extended periods without food.

- Long-term adherence can be challenging, and there's potential risk for nutrient deficiencies if not done thoughtfully.

Impact on Lifespan and Healthspan

While both IF and CR have shown potential lifespan-extending benefits in various animal models, their exact impacts on human longevity remain an area of active research. Both approaches seem to enhance healthspan, with potential benefits including reduced inflammation, improved metabolic health, and better cardiovascular outcomes.

Concluding Thoughts

Intermittent Fasting and Caloric Restriction, while sharing the overarching theme of food limitation, have distinct methodologies, physiological effects, and practical considerations. The choice between them (or a combination thereof) depends on individual preferences, lifestyle, health goals, and, importantly, how one's body responds. As always, before initiating significant dietary changes, it's advisable to consult with healthcare professionals to ensure the approach is safe and appropriate for one's specific circumstances.

How these approaches affect the body and longevity

Intermittent Fasting (IF) and Caloric Restriction (CR) have made waves in the health and wellness sphere, in part due to their potential longevity-enhancing properties. The mechanisms by which they influence the body and, possibly, the duration of life are rooted in a blend of metabolic, cellular, and hormonal changes. This section elucidates how IF and CR affect the body and their associated implications for longevity.

Metabolic Shifts

1. Intermittent Fasting:

- **Glycogen Depletion**: Prolonged fasting drains the liver's glycogen reserves, prompting the body to shift towards burning fat, a process culminating in mild ketosis.

- **Insulin Sensitivity**: Regular fasting intervals can bolster insulin sensitivity, facilitating better blood sugar management.

2. Caloric Restriction:

- **Metabolic Slowdown**: With consistent caloric deficits, the body may reduce its metabolic rate as an adaptive measure to conserve energy.

- **Enhanced Fat Oxidation**: A caloric deficit often necessitates increased fat metabolism to meet energy requirements.

Cellular and Molecular Changes

1. Intermittent Fasting:

- **Autophagy**: One of the most lauded cellular benefits of IF is autophagy, a cellular "clean-up" process where cells dismantle damaged components, potentially enhancing cellular longevity.

- **Stress Resistance**: IF can foster cellular resilience against oxidative stress, potentially attenuating aging's cellular wear and tear.

2. Caloric Restriction:

- **DNA Repair**: Reduced caloric intake has been linked to improved DNA repair mechanisms, potentially curtailing the accumulation of mutations that might drive aging.

- **Protein Homeostasis**: CR promotes more efficient protein synthesis and recycling, fostering healthier cellular function.

Hormonal Adjustments

3. Intermittent Fasting:

- **Growth Hormone Release:** Fasting periods can spur episodic surges in growth hormone, which plays a role in fat metabolism and muscle maintenance.

- **Modified Leptin and Ghrelin Levels:** These hunger hormones might adjust with IF, influencing appetite and satiety signals.

4. Caloric Restriction:

- **Reduced IGF-1:** A consistent caloric deficit can decrease Insulin-like Growth Factor-1 levels, a molecule associated with various aging processes and age-related diseases.

- **Optimized Insulin Dynamics:** Just as with IF, CR can promote improved insulin sensitivity.

Longevity Implications

Both IF and CR have exhibited longevity benefits in a spectrum of animal models, from worms and flies to mice. The longevity perks are believed to stem from the interplay of metabolic recalibrations, cellular health enhancement, and hormonal adjustments, which together may stave off age-associated physiological decline.

For humans, the precise lifespan-extending benefits remain an open question, albeit there's mounting evidence that both IF and CR significantly boost healthspan. This means that while we might not have definitive proof of added years to life, there's robust evidence for added life to years.

Benefits observed include:

- **Reduced Inflammation:** Chronic inflammation is a consistent accomplice in aging and many age-related diseases. Both IF and CR can dampen inflammatory processes.
- **Cardiovascular Health:** Enhanced lipid profiles, blood pressure regulation, and arterial health have been observed with both approaches.

- **Neuroprotective Effects:** Both IF and CR seem to offer protection against neurodegenerative processes, potentially through enhanced autophagy, reduced oxidative stress, and bolstered neuronal plasticity.

Concluding Thoughts

Intermittent Fasting and Caloric Restriction, while differing in their methodologies, harbor substantial overlap in their health and potential longevity benefits. Their interlinked metabolic, cellular, and hormonal shifts offer a compelling argument for the inclusion of some form of dietary restriction in the quest for a prolonged, health-rich life. As our understanding evolves, it's hopeful we'll gain clearer insights into optimizing these strategies for the human lifespan.

Considerations for those interested in trying these methods

Embarking on a journey of Intermittent Fasting (IF) or Caloric Restriction (CR) demands more than just an informed understanding of their theoretical benefits. Practical considerations, potential challenges, and individual variations play crucial roles in determining the success and sustainability of these dietary approaches. This section offers guidance for individuals contemplating these methods.

Understand Your "Why"

Before diving into IF or CR, it's vital to understand your motivations.

- **Health or Longevity:** Some are driven by the desire for better health outcomes, while others might be chasing the potential longevity benefits.
- **Weight Management:** Others might be primarily interested in weight loss or metabolic health improvements.

Clearly delineating your goals helps tailor the approach and set realistic expectations.

Assess Your Current Health Status

1. **Medical Conditions**: Individuals with certain conditions like diabetes or heart issues should approach IF or CR with caution and under medical supervision.

2. **Mental Health**: Those with a history of eating disorders or related psychological conditions should consider whether these approaches are appropriate and safe.

Start Slowly

Especially for beginners, drastic changes can be overwhelming and counterproductive.

1. **Intermittent Fasting**: Instead of diving into a stringent 16/8 regime, one might start with a 12/12 pattern, gradually extending the fasting window.

2. **Caloric Restriction**: A sudden, significant reduction in calorie intake can be jarring. Consider a moderate reduction initially and adjust based on how your body responds.

Monitor Nutrient Intake

Restricting eating windows or calories shouldn't equate to nutrient deprivation.

1. **Intermittent Fasting**: Ensure that during your eating windows, you're consuming nutritionally dense foods to meet your body's requirements.

2. **Caloric Restriction**: It becomes even more crucial to maximize nutrient density per calorie, ensuring you're getting essential vitamins, minerals, and other nutrients despite eating less.

Stay Hydrated

Both IF and CR can alter hydration needs and dynamics.

- **Drink Ample Water:** Especially during fasting periods in IF, drinking water can also help manage hunger pangs.
- **Electrolytes:** Extended fasting or significant calorie reductions may necessitate attention to electrolyte intake to prevent imbalances.

Listen to Your Body

While structured guidelines can be helpful, individual responses vary.

- **Adjust Based on Feedback:** If you're feeling overly fatigued, dizzy, or experiencing other adverse reactions, it might indicate a need for modifications.
- **Flexibility:** It's okay to adjust fasting windows or calorie intake based on daily activities, energy needs, or special occasions.

Educate Yourself on Potential Side Effects

Both IF and CR come with potential side effects, especially during the adaptation phase.

- **Common Side Effects:** These might include headaches, dizziness, irritability, or fatigue.
- **Mitigation:** Often, these side effects wane as the body adapts. However, understanding them in advance can prevent undue alarm and provide strategies for mitigation.

Consider Social and Lifestyle Implications

1. **Social Gatherings:** If your social life revolves around meals, IF might necessitate planning to accommodate your chosen eating windows.

2. **Workout Regimens:** Those with strenuous exercise routines might need to time their eating windows or caloric intake to fuel their workouts effectively.

Seek Support and Information

- **Community**: Online forums, local groups, or even friends and family on similar journeys can provide support, insights, and camaraderie.

- **Stay Updated**: Nutritional science is ever-evolving. Regularly update your knowledge to ensure you're making informed decisions.

Conclusion

Embracing Intermittent Fasting or Caloric Restriction can be a transformative experience, but it demands an informed and mindful approach. By understanding potential challenges, tailoring strategies to personal circumstances, and consistently listening to one's body, individuals can optimize these methods for health, well-being, and potential longevity benefits.

Chapter 8:
Blue Zones – Lessons from the Longest Lived

Introduction to the Blue Zones and their dietary patterns

In the quest to understand the secrets of longevity, researchers have turned their attention to specific regions around the world where people live exceptionally long, healthy lives. These regions, termed "Blue Zones," have been the subject of intense scrutiny, not only for the longevity of their inhabitants but also for the quality of life these individuals enjoy in their later years. This section introduces the concept of Blue Zones and delves into the dietary patterns that might contribute to their residents' impressive lifespans.

What are Blue Zones?

The term "Blue Zones" was popularized by Dan Buettner, a National Geographic Fellow and author, who, along with a team of demographers and scientists, identified five regions where people live statistically longer:

1. **Okinawa, Japan:** Often recognized for its elderly female population, where many live to be over 100.

2. **Sardinia, Italy:** Particularly the mountainous region of Barbagia, known for its high number of centenarian men.

3. **Nicoya Peninsula, Costa Rica:** A region characterized by its residents' zest for life well into old age.

4. **Ikaria, Greece:** An island in the Aegean Sea, distinguished by its low rates of middle age mortality and a high number of residents living into their 90s.

5. **Loma Linda, California**: A community of Seventh-day Adventists who outlive their North American counterparts by several years.

Common Dietary Patterns

While each Blue Zone has its unique cultural and dietary practices, several commonalities emerge when examining their eating habits.

1. **Plant-Predominant Diets**: All Blue Zones emphasize plant-based foods. Fruits, vegetables, legumes, whole grains, and nuts form the majority of their dietary intake.

2. **Limited Meat Consumption**: Meat, especially red meat, is consumed infrequently and in moderation—often just a few times a month and in small portions.

3. **Whole Foods**: Highly processed foods are rare. Instead, fresh, seasonal, and locally-sourced items dominate.

4. **Healthy Fats**: Olive oil in Ikaria and Sardinia, or the omega-3 rich fish in Okinawa, contribute to a diet rich in beneficial fats.

5. **Moderate Alcohol**: Except for Loma Linda, moderate alcohol consumption, particularly wine, is common. In Sardinia and Ikaria, for instance, red wine is enjoyed with meals and friends.

6. **Hydration**: Fresh water, herbal teas, and natural beverages are preferred over sugary drinks or excessive caffeine.

7. **Mindful Eating**: Beyond just the type of food, how it's consumed matters. Eating with family, savoring meals slowly, and ceasing to eat when 80% full (a practice known as *Hara Hachi Bu* in Okinawa) are integral to their eating habits.

The Broader Picture

While diet undoubtedly plays a crucial role in the longevity seen in these regions, it's essential to note that it's just one piece of the puzzle. Lifestyle factors, such as physical activity, strong social connections, stress management, and a sense of purpose, also significantly contribute to the health and vitality seen in Blue Zones. The interplay between diet, lifestyle, and perhaps even genetics creates a synergistic effect, leading to the impressive longevity outcomes observed.

Conclusion

The Blue Zones serve as living laboratories, offering insights into the dietary and lifestyle practices that can promote longevity. Their emphasis on plant-based, whole foods, coupled with a holistic approach to well-being, provides valuable lessons for those seeking not just longer, but more fulfilling lives. As we delve deeper into each Blue Zone in subsequent sections, we'll uncover more specifics and the nuanced differences that make each region unique.

Shared dietary traits among Blue Zones

The Blue Zones—regions renowned for their exceptional longevity—hold invaluable lessons for those keen on understanding the dietary patterns linked to long and healthy lives. While each Blue Zone boasts distinct culinary traditions influenced by local resources, culture, and history, there are striking dietary commonalities. These shared traits offer insight into the core principles that may be at the heart of their longevity success.

1. Emphasis on Plant-Based Foods

All Blue Zones demonstrate a predominant reliance on plants:

- **Legumes:** Beans, lentils, chickpeas, and other legumes are staple proteins. In Nicoya, black beans reign supreme, while in Sardinia, fava beans and chickpeas are popular.
- **Vegetables:** From the bitter melon of Okinawa to the wild greens of Ikaria, vegetables are consumed in abundance.
- **Fruits:** Seasonal fruits, whether it's the citrus in Okinawa or the figs in Sardinia, are a regular treat.
- **Whole Grains:** Be it the whole wheat bread in Ikaria or maize tortillas in Nicoya, whole grains provide essential carbohydrates.

2. Limited Consumption of Meat

Meat plays a secondary role:

- **Occasional Serving**: Many Blue Zones residents eat meat but often only a few times a month.
- **Portion Control**: When consumed, portion sizes are generally modest—typically the size of a deck of cards.

3. Favoring Fish

While meat is limited, fish often finds its way onto the plate:

- **Small, Local Fish**: Rather than large predatory fish, smaller varieties, often locally caught, are favored. For instance, Okinawans might eat fish like mackerel, rich in omega-3 fatty acids.
- **Frequency**: Some zones, especially those near water, incorporate fish into meals a few times a week.

4. Whole, Unprocessed Foods

Processed foods are conspicuously absent:

- **Minimally Processed**: The majority of what's consumed is close to its natural state.
- **Seasonal and Fresh**: There's an emphasis on eating foods in their season. This not only provides variety but ensures peak nutrition.
- **Home Cooking**: Prepared meals at home from scratch are the norm, allowing control over ingredients and methods.

5. Healthy Fats, Not Avoided

Beneficial fats are embraced:

- **Olive Oil**: Regions like Ikaria and Sardinia liberally use olive oil, a source of heart-healthy monounsaturated fats.
- **Nuts and Seeds**: These are regular snacks or additions to dishes. Loma Linda's Seventh-day Adventists, for example, regularly consume a variety of nuts.

6. Dairy in Moderation

Where dairy is consumed, it's specific and often fermented:

- **Sheep and Goat Dairy**: In places like Sardinia, sheep and goat milk products, which can be easier to digest than cow's milk, are more prevalent.
- **Fermented Products**: Items like yogurt or cheese, which contain beneficial probiotics, are favored.

7. Limited Sugar and Sweets

Sugary treats are infrequent and savored:

- **Natural Sweeteners**: Honey, especially in places like Ikaria, might be used.
- **Celebration Foods**: Desserts and sweets are often reserved for special occasions rather than daily indulgence.

8. Hydration and Moderate Alcohol

Pure, simple hydration is prioritized:

- **Water**: The primary beverage across all zones.
- **Moderate Alcohol**: With the exception of Loma Linda, moderate alcohol, especially wine, is consumed, often with meals.

9. Herbs and Spices

Many regions use herbs not only for flavor but potential health benefits:

- **Turmeric in Okinawa, rosemary in Ikaria**, and **oregano in Sardinia** are just a few examples.

Conclusion

The dietary threads running through the Blue Zones weave a tapestry of insights. A focus on whole, plant-based foods; limited meat; an embrace of beneficial fats; and a mindful approach to eating emerge as shared tenets. These dietary choices, embedded within broader lifestyles of physical activity, strong community ties, and purpose, seem to create a synergy that pushes the boundaries of human longevity.

How culture and lifestyle complement dietary habits

While the Blue Zones offer profound insights into dietary patterns conducive to longevity, it's crucial to recognize that diet is just one piece of a multifaceted mosaic. The tapestry of longevity in these regions is intricately woven with threads of culture, tradition, and lifestyle. These elements, in tandem with nutritional habits, form a holistic approach to life that seems to favor both lifespan and healthspan.

1. Physical Activity Integrated into Daily Life

In Blue Zones, there's no distinct delineation between exercise and daily life. Physical activity is seamlessly integrated into everyday routines:

- **Natural Movement:** From the fishermen of Ikaria to the garden-tending elders of Okinawa, routine tasks inherently involve movement.
- **No Gyms:** The idea of scheduled gym sessions is foreign. Instead, natural landscapes, from the mountains of Sardinia to the beaches of Nicoya, serve as the backdrop for physical exertion.

2. Strong Social Connections

Community and connection are central tenets of life in Blue Zones:

- **Close-Knit Communities:** Whether it's the *moai* groups of Okinawa, where individuals forge lifelong social bonds, or the tight-knit villages of Sardinia, social connections are deep-rooted.
- **Multigenerational Interaction:** Elderly individuals aren't relegated to the periphery. They often live with family, playing an active role in community life, which instills a sense of purpose and combats loneliness.

3. Mindfulness and Stress Reduction

A common thread in Blue Zones is the emphasis on managing stress and embracing the present:

- **Natural Breaks:** The *siestas* in Ikaria or the Seventh-day Adventist's Sabbath in Loma Linda serve as periodic respites from daily hustle.
- **Mindful Practices:** Whether it's the traditional tea ceremonies in Okinawa or meditation sessions in Loma Linda, mindfulness practices are integrated into life.

4. Sense of Purpose

Having a reason to wake up in the morning—a clear purpose—seems to be a shared sentiment:

- **Ikigai and Plan de Vida:** While the Okinawans call it *Ikigai* and the Nicoyans term it *Plan de Vida*, both essentially mean having a sense of purpose in life.
- **Continued Roles:** Elders in these regions often continue to contribute to communities, whether through imparting wisdom, taking care of grandchildren, or even working in fields or businesses.

5. Cultural Celebrations and Traditions

Cultural festivities, often revolving around food, play a pivotal role:

- **Seasonal Feasts:** Be it the grape harvest in Sardinia or local festivals in Okinawa, these celebrations emphasize communal eating, dancing, and merriment.
- **Local Traditions:** Each zone has unique traditions—like the Sardinian *canto a tenore* or the Okinawan *Eisa* dance—that strengthen community bonds and promote well-being.

6. Attitude Toward Food

Beyond the ingredients, the approach to food is deeply cultural:

- **Mindful Consumption:** Practices like the aforementioned *Hara Hachi Bu* in Okinawa instill a mindful approach to eating.

- **Communal Meals**: Dining is often a communal affair, emphasizing connection and conversation over rushed meals.

Conclusion

Dietary patterns in the Blue Zones, while essential, do not operate in isolation. They're part of a holistic lifestyle that emphasizes community, purpose, physical activity, and mindfulness. This interwoven approach suggests that the quest for longevity isn't about any single magic bullet, but rather a symphony of factors playing harmoniously together. To truly glean the secrets of the Blue Zones, one must appreciate this synergy and recognize that food, while central, is just one note in a beautiful melody.

Chapter 9:
The Role of Supplements and Longevity

Popular supplements and their impact on health and lifespan

In our modern age, the allure of supplements—a quick, concentrated boost of nutrients—has never been stronger. Amidst the promise of enhanced health, energy, and lifespan, a deluge of capsules, powders, and liquids beckon consumers. Yet, does the science support the claims? Here, we explore popular supplements and their purported impact on health and longevity.

1. Vitamin D

Often dubbed the "sunshine vitamin" due to its synthesis in our skin upon sun exposure, Vitamin D is crucial for bone health, immune function, and more:

- **Benefits**: Assists in calcium absorption, supporting bone health. Has roles in immune modulation and may reduce inflammation.
- **Studies**: Some research links Vitamin D deficiency with increased mortality, especially in older adults. However, it's unclear if supplementation can significantly alter lifespan for those with adequate levels.

2. Omega-3 Fatty Acids

Derived mainly from fish oil, these fats are hailed for their anti-inflammatory properties:

- **Benefits**: Supports cardiovascular health, reduces inflammation, and may boost cognitive health.
- **Studies**: Regular consumption of fish is associated with reduced risk of chronic diseases. However, the benefits of omega-3 supplements, especially in already healthy individuals, remain contested.

3. Resveratrol

Found in red wine, grapes, and some berries, resveratrol gained fame as a potential longevity booster:

- **Benefits**: Antioxidant and anti-inflammatory effects. Has been shown to extend lifespan in some animal models.
- **Studies**: Human studies are limited. While it has potential cardiovascular and anti-cancer benefits, its direct impact on human lifespan is yet to be conclusively established.

4. Probiotics

Touted for gut health, these are live beneficial bacteria:

- **Benefits**: Can aid in digestion, enhance gut microbiome diversity, and boost immune function.
- **Studies**: A healthy gut microbiome is associated with reduced risk of several diseases. Probiotics can be beneficial in specific scenarios (like antibiotic-induced gut disruption) but their universal longevity benefits need more exploration.

5. Vitamin C

Popularly associated with immune support, it's an essential antioxidant:

- **Benefits**: Supports immune function, aids in collagen production, and acts as an antioxidant.
- **Studies**: While severe deficiency (scurvy) is detrimental, there's scant evidence that high doses extend lifespan. Some studies suggest it may reduce the severity and duration of colds.

6. Coenzyme Q10 (CoQ10)

A natural compound with roles in energy production:

- **Benefits**: Essential for cellular energy production, acts as an antioxidant, and supports heart health.
- **Studies**: Might be beneficial for specific conditions like heart failure. As a general longevity booster, the evidence is mixed.

7. Turmeric/Curcumin

An age-old spice with anti-inflammatory and antioxidant properties:

- **Benefits**: Can reduce inflammation, possibly support brain and joint health.
- **Studies**: While the anti-inflammatory effects are well-documented, longevity-specific research in humans is limited.

Conclusion

The world of supplements is vast, promising, and at times, perplexing. While certain supplements offer clear health benefits, especially when addressing deficiencies or specific conditions, their role as universal longevity boosters is less clear-cut. It's always essential to approach supplementation judiciously, consulting with healthcare professionals. Ultimately, no supplement can replace the holistic benefits of a balanced diet, active lifestyle, and overall well-being.

The debate around the necessity of supplements

As the supplement industry burgeons, so too does the debate surrounding their necessity. Are these pills and powders a health panacea, or merely modern-day snake oil? Dive into the contentious dialogue and discern fact from fiction.

1. The Pro-Supplement Argument

For many, supplements appear as a beacon of hope in an often nutritionally inadequate world:

- **Addressing Deficiencies**: Modern diets, often dominated by processed foods, can be deficient in essential nutrients. Supplements offer a straightforward remedy.
- **Bioavailability Boost**: Some argue that supplements, especially in liquid or sublingual forms, can be more readily absorbed than nutrients from food.

- **Targeted Interventions**: Individuals with specific health conditions or concerns can find targeted relief with supplements, like iron for anemia or probiotics post-antibiotics.

2. The Anti-Supplement Stance

For every proponent, there's a skeptic questioning the widespread adoption of supplementation:

- **Whole Foods First**: Many argue that nutrients are best sourced from whole foods, which offer a synergistic blend of vitamins, minerals, and phytochemicals.
- **Overconsumption Risks**: Unlike whole foods, which naturally regulate consumption, it's easy to overdose on supplements, potentially causing harm.
- **Lack of Regulation**: The supplement industry, especially in places like the U.S., isn't rigorously regulated. This means quality, purity, and efficacy can vary drastically.

3. Science's Take

The scientific community provides a more nuanced perspective:

- **Case-by-Case Basis**: Most researchers agree that supplements can be beneficial, but their necessity should be assessed individually. While a Vitamin D supplement might be vital for someone in sun-deprived regions, it might be superfluous for another living in sunnier climes.
- **Beyond Basic Nutrients**: The debate gets murkier with non-essential supplements. While a magnesium supplement might aid sleep for some, the jury is still out on adaptogens like ashwagandha or luxury supplements like pearl powder.
- **Interaction with Medications**: There's growing concern about how supplements interact with prescription medications. For example, St. John's Wort, a popular herbal supplement, can interfere with the efficacy of birth control pills and certain antidepressants.

4. The Role of Marketing

A significant portion of the debate can be traced back to the powerful supplement marketing machine:

- **Miracle Claims**: Supplemented by celebrity endorsements and influencer marketing, some supplements are touted as cure-alls, from reversing aging to boosting intelligence. These claims often lack rigorous scientific backing.

- **Selective Science**: Some companies cherry-pick studies, highlighting the positive while ignoring contradictory evidence.

5. Consumer Perception and Behavior

The public's perception plays a crucial role in fueling the debate:

- **Quick Fixes**: In a world seeking instant solutions, supplements often appear as an attractive shortcut to health.

- **Placebo Effect**: For many, just the act of taking a supplement can induce a placebo effect, making them feel better, irrespective of any physiological impact.

Conclusion

The debate around the necessity of supplements is unlikely to be settled soon. While they can undeniably play a role in health—filling nutritional gaps, aiding specific conditions—their universal adoption as daily must-haves is more contentious. It underscores the importance of personalized health approaches, where individual needs, not generalized marketing claims, dictate choices. As with many health dilemmas, a balanced perspective—prioritizing whole foods, using supplements judiciously, and consulting professionals—is likely the optimal path.

Best practices for supplement intake

In the vast sea of supplements, with its enticing promises and potential pitfalls, how does one navigate safely? Here, we outline best practices for supplement intake, ensuring you reap benefits while minimizing risks.

1. Determine the Need

Before introducing any supplement into your regimen:

- **Medical Evaluation**: Always start with a thorough check-up. Blood tests can pinpoint deficiencies, guiding targeted supplementation.
- **Symptom Analysis**: If you're experiencing symptoms like fatigue, hair loss, or brittle nails, they might indicate a specific nutrient deficiency.

2. Quality Over Quantity

Not all supplements are created equal:

- **Research Brands**: Look for brands with a reputation for purity and efficacy. Reputable ones often undergo third-party testing.
- **Avoid Fillers**: Many supplements contain unnecessary fillers, binders, or artificial colors. Aim for products with minimal additives.

3. Educate Yourself

Understanding what you're consuming is paramount:

- **Read Labels**: Familiarize yourself with active ingredients, dosages, and any other compounds in the supplement.
- **Expiry Date**: Nutrients can degrade over time. Ensure you're consuming supplements well before their expiration date.

4. Right Dosage

More doesn't always mean better:

- **Follow Guidelines**: Stick to the recommended daily dosages, unless advised otherwise by a healthcare professional.
- **Beware of Megadoses**: While certain nutrients are harmless in large quantities, others can be toxic. For instance, excessive vitamin A intake can lead to nausea, dizziness, and even hair loss.

5. Consider Timing and Synergy

When and how you take supplements can influence their effectiveness:

- **With or Without Food:** Some vitamins, like Vitamin E and D, are fat-soluble and better absorbed with meals. Others, like B vitamins, might be best on an empty stomach.
- **Synergy:** Certain nutrients work better together. Calcium and Vitamin D are a classic pairing, with the latter enhancing the absorption of the former.

6. Stay Updated with Research

The world of nutritional science is ever-evolving:

- **Latest Studies:** What's deemed beneficial today might be debunked tomorrow. Stay updated with recent research.
- **Consult Professionals:** Regularly consult nutritionists or dieticians. They can offer insights into the latest findings and tailor recommendations.

7. Listen to Your Body

While empirical evidence is vital, personal experience shouldn't be discounted:

- **Side Effects:** If you notice any adverse reactions post-supplementation—rashes, digestive issues, or palpitations—cease intake and consult a doctor.
- **Positive Outcomes:** Conversely, if a supplement significantly enhances your well-being and has scientific backing, it's likely a good fit.

8. Interactions with Medications

Many are unaware of how supplements can interfere with medications:

- **Provide Full Lists:** Whenever you're prescribed a new medication, ensure the prescribing physician knows about all your supplements.

- **Common Culprits**: Some supplements are notorious for interactions. For example, Ginkgo Biloba might increase bleeding risks if taken with blood thinners.

9. Re-evaluate Periodically

Your nutritional needs can shift:

- **Changing Life Stages**: Pregnancy, aging, or specific health conditions can alter your nutrient requirements.
- **Regular Check-ups**: Annual evaluations can help adjust supplement regimens, adding or subtracting based on current needs.

Conclusion

Supplement intake, when approached with care and knowledge, can be a boon to health. But it's essential to tread wisely, balancing the allure of promising pills with evidence-based, individualized choices. By adhering to these best practices, you can harness the benefits of supplements, bolstering health and potentially even longevity.

Chapter 10:
Pitfalls of Modern Diets

The rise of processed foods and their impact on health

In the grand tapestry of human evolution, processed foods are a recent blip, yet their dominance in modern diets is indisputable. From instant noodles to frozen pizzas, they promise convenience, but at what cost? Delve into the rise of processed foods and their multifaceted impact on health.

1. A Historical Perspective

Our ancestors' diets were largely dictated by seasons, availability, and geographical location:

- **Whole Foods:** Most consumed foods were unprocessed or minimally processed, like fruits, vegetables, grains, and lean meats.

- **Industrial Revolution:** With technological advancements, the late 19th and early 20th centuries saw the dawn of modern food processing—canned foods, pasteurization, and refined sugars and flours.

2. The Allure of Processed Foods

The rapid proliferation of processed foods can be attributed to several factors:

- **Convenience:** In our fast-paced world, quick meals are attractive. Processed foods, with their extended shelf life and minimal preparation time, fit the bill.

- **Cost:** Often cheaper than fresh produce, especially in urban settings, they appeal to budget-conscious consumers.

- **Taste & Marketing:** High in sugars, salts, and fats, processed foods cater to our innate taste preferences, amplified by aggressive marketing.

3. Nutritional Downfalls

While they might satiate taste buds, nutritionally, processed foods often fall short:

- **Empty Calories**: Laden with sugars and unhealthy fats, they provide calories without the corresponding nutritional value.
- **Reduced Vitamins & Minerals**: Processing can strip foods of essential nutrients. For example, refining grains removes the nutrient-rich bran and germ.
- **Additives & Preservatives**: To enhance flavor and prolong shelf life, a plethora of chemicals are added, some of which raise health concerns.

4. Health Implications

The consistent consumption of processed foods has been linked to a slew of health issues:

- **Obesity**: High in calories and low in satiety, these foods can lead to overeating and weight gain.
- **Heart Diseases**: Trans fats, prevalent in many processed foods, are associated with increased heart disease risk.
- **Type 2 Diabetes**: Excessive sugar and unhealthy fats can exacerbate insulin resistance.
- **Digestive Issues**: Low in fiber, many processed foods can disrupt digestive health, leading to constipation or other gastrointestinal problems.

5. Mental Health Connections

Emerging research indicates that the repercussions aren't limited to physical health:

- **Mood Fluctuations**: Excessive sugar intake can lead to blood sugar spikes and crashes, affecting mood.
- **Long-term Impacts**: Diets high in processed foods have been linked to increased depression and anxiety risks.

6. Socioeconomic and Environmental Concerns

Beyond individual health, the rise of processed foods poses broader challenges:

- **Economic Disparities**: In many areas, healthy foods are pricier and less accessible than processed alternatives, perpetuating health disparities.
- **Environmental Strain**: The mass production of processed foods often involves intensive farming, excessive water use, and significant waste, amplifying their environmental footprint.

7. Finding Balance

While the drawbacks are evident, it's unrealistic to expect a complete exodus from processed foods:

- **Informed Choices**: Not all processed foods are detrimental. For instance, frozen fruits or canned legumes can be nutritious if free from added sugars or excessive salt.
- **Limiting Harmful Variants**: Aim to reduce foods high in trans fats, added sugars, and sodium.

Conclusion

The rise of processed foods reflects a broader societal shift towards convenience and speed. However, with this convenience comes a health cost, evident in the global uptick in diet-related diseases. Recognizing the pitfalls of processed foods and making informed dietary choices is pivotal, ensuring that convenience doesn't compromise longevity.

The dangers of excessive sugar, salt, and unhealthy fats

A key reason behind the health detriments of many modern diets is the abundant presence of three culprits: sugar, salt, and unhealthy fats. Individually, each poses distinct health risks, but collectively, their ubiquity in processed foods forms a trifecta of dietary concerns.

1. Sugar: The Sweet Deception

At first glance, sugar seems harmless—after all, it's derived from plants like sugar cane or beets. However, the health implications of excessive sugar intake are manifold.

- **Caloric Density:** Sugar is calorie-dense. Consuming foods high in added sugars can lead to inadvertent calorie overloads, contributing to weight gain.
- **Insulin Resistance and Diabetes**: Constant sugar influx can overburden the body's insulin response. Over time, this may result in insulin resistance, a precursor to Type 2 diabetes.
- **Heart Health:** High sugar intake has been linked to increased risks of heart diseases. It can raise blood pressure, increase chronic inflammation, and elevate triglyceride levels.
- **Tooth Decay:** Sugar provides an ideal breeding ground for bacteria in our mouths, leading to cavities.

2. Salt: Beyond the Shaker

While sodium—an element in salt—is essential for nerve and muscle functions, its excessive intake is problematic.

- **Hypertension (High Blood Pressure):** High salt intake can cause the body to retain water, putting additional pressure on blood vessels and the heart, leading to hypertension—a major risk factor for heart diseases and stroke.
- **Kidney Function:** Overburdened by the need to filter excessive sodium, kidneys can be adversely affected in the long run.
- **Osteoporosis**: High salt diets might increase calcium loss through urine, potentially weakening bones and increasing osteoporosis risk.

3. Unhealthy Fats: The Good, the Bad, and the Ugly

All fats aren't created equal. While some fats (like those from avocados or nuts) are beneficial, others can be detrimental to health.

- **Saturated Fats:** Found primarily in animal products like meat and dairy, high intake can increase LDL (bad) cholesterol levels, elevating heart disease risk.

- **Trans Fats**: These are industrially produced fats, introduced to increase the shelf life of processed foods. They not only raise LDL cholesterol but also reduce HDL (good) cholesterol. The World Health Organization aims to eliminate trans fats from the global food supply due to their profound negative health impacts.

4. Collective Implications

While each of these dietary elements poses individual risks, their cumulative presence in many processed foods amplifies potential harm.

- **Obesity Epidemic**: Sugary, salty, fat-laden foods can be addictive, encouraging overconsumption and contributing to the global obesity crisis.
- **Diet-Related Diseases**: The confluence of these elements has been implicated in the surge of diet-related diseases, from cardiovascular diseases to certain cancers.

5. A Word on Addictive Patterns

Research indicates that foods high in sugar, salt, and fats can activate reward centers in the brain, similar to certain drugs. Over time, this can encourage compulsive eating behaviors.

6. Finding Moderation

While eliminating sugar, salt, and fats is unrealistic (and unhealthy, given that they do have roles in bodily functions):

- **Reading Labels**: Check product labels for added sugars, sodium content, and unhealthy fats. Opt for alternatives with lower amounts of these ingredients.
- **Whole Foods**: Prioritize whole, unprocessed foods, which naturally have a healthier balance of these elements.

Conclusion

The prominence of sugar, salt, and unhealthy fats in many modern diets underpins the health challenges of our times. Recognizing their risks and making conscious dietary choices can help navigate the pitfalls of modern diets, ensuring optimal health and longevity.

Strategies to avoid common dietary pitfalls

In a world filled with tempting, calorie-laden delicacies, steering clear of dietary pitfalls can seem daunting. However, by adopting a few mindful strategies, one can navigate the modern food landscape adeptly, optimizing both health and pleasure from meals.

1. Educate Yourself: Know the Culprits

Before you can avoid the pitfalls, you must recognize them.

- **Reading Labels:** Familiarize yourself with nutritional labels. Understand terms like trans fats, added sugars, and sodium. This knowledge is the first step towards making informed choices.
- **Stay Updated:** Nutritional science is evolving. Regularly educate yourself on the latest research about dietary health.

2. Cook More, Order Less

Home-cooked meals are often more nutritious and less calorie-dense than restaurant offerings.

- **Recipe Exploration:** Dive into the world of healthy recipes. Cooking can be a therapeutic and creative process.
- **Plan Ahead:** Batch cook meals during weekends. Store in portions for a hassle-free week ahead.

3. Mindful Eating: Savor Each Bite

The pace and mindfulness with which you eat can profoundly affect your consumption.

- **Slow Down:** It takes the brain about 20 minutes to register fullness. Eating slowly can help you recognize when you're satiated.
- **Distraction-Free:** Eat away from screens and workspaces. This fosters mindfulness, making overeating less likely.

4. Hydration: The Forgotten Element

Often, our bodies confuse thirst with hunger.

- **Regular Hydration:** Ensure you're drinking sufficient water throughout the day. This can keep 'hunger' in check.
- **Begin with Water:** Start each meal with a glass of water. It primes the stomach and can moderate food intake.

5. Be Proactive When Eating Out

Eating out doesn't mean you must surrender to dietary pitfalls.

- **Research:** Check the restaurant's menu in advance. Look for healthier options.
- **Beware of Liquid Calories:** Sodas and certain alcoholic beverages can be calorie bombs. Opt for water, herbal teas, or simple beverages.
- **Portion Control:** Restaurant servings are often oversized. Consider sharing dishes or packing half for later.

6. Prioritize Whole Foods

A diet centered around whole foods naturally limits unhealthy additives.

- **Shop the Periphery:** In many supermarkets, the outer aisles house fresh produce, while the inner aisles contain more processed items.
- **Limit Refined Carbohydrates:** Swap white bread and pasta for whole grain alternatives. They're more nutritious and satiating.

7. Moderation Over Deprivation

It's okay to indulge occasionally. The key is balance.

- **80-20 Rule:** Aim to eat healthily 80% of the time. This leaves room for occasional treats.
- **Listen to Your Body:** Recognize genuine cravings versus fleeting desires. Grant yourself the occasional indulgence without guilt.

8. Stay Active

While this isn't a direct dietary strategy, physical activity can help regulate appetite and boost metabolism.

- **Regular Movement**: Find activities you love. From yoga to dancing to running, there's something for everyone.
- **Break the Sedentary Cycle**: If your job involves prolonged sitting, set regular alarms to get up and stretch or walk.

9. Cultivate a Supportive Community

Dietary habits can be socially influenced.

- **Find Your Tribe**: Connect with like-minded individuals, be it online or in local communities. They can offer encouragement, tips, and accountability.
- **Educate Loved Ones**: Share what you learn about nutrition with family and friends. This can foster collective health awareness.

Conclusion

Avoiding dietary pitfalls in the modern world is more about mindfulness and moderation than sheer willpower. By integrating these strategies into daily life, one can enjoy the pleasures of diverse cuisines while ensuring longevity and robust health.

Chapter 11:
Integrating Diet with Other Longevity Practices

The importance of exercise and its synergy with diet

In the quest for longevity and optimal health, two critical components stand out: diet and exercise. While both are individually potent, their combined effects create a synergy that can amplify the benefits of each, leading to enhanced well-being and increased life expectancy.

1. Bi-directional Benefits of Diet and Exercise

When we consume a nutritious diet, we provide our bodies with the essential fuel it needs. This energy allows for more effective workouts, helping the body to recover and rebuild faster post-exercise.

Conversely, regular exercise enhances metabolism, aids in effective nutrient absorption, and can help regulate appetite. This ensures that the nutritious foods consumed are optimally utilized, curbing excessive caloric intake.

2. Combined Role in Weight Management

Achieving and maintaining a healthy weight is crucial for longevity. Here's where the synergy between diet and exercise plays a vital role:

- **Caloric Balance:** While diet primarily determines caloric intake, exercise helps in caloric expenditure. Balancing these two is key to weight management.
- **Body Composition:** While weight loss can be achieved through diet alone, incorporating strength training ensures the preservation of muscle mass, leading to a more favorable body composition.

3. Enhanced Cardiovascular Health

Heart health is foundational to longevity.

- **Diet's Role**: Nutritious diets rich in omega-3 fatty acids, fiber, and antioxidants can lower bad cholesterol levels, reduce blood pressure, and decrease inflammation.
- **Exercise's Role**: Regular cardiovascular activities, like running or swimming, strengthen the heart muscle, improve circulation, and increase lung capacity.

Together, these lifestyle choices create a fortified defense against cardiovascular diseases.

4. Strengthened Immune System

Diet and exercise have been shown to bolster the immune system's defense mechanisms.

- **Nutritional Boost**: Vitamins and minerals, like vitamin C, vitamin E, and zinc, are essential for immune function. A balanced diet ensures a regular supply.
- **Exercise Impact**: Physical activity can promote good circulation, allowing immune cells to move efficiently throughout the body, heightening their effectiveness.

5. Improved Digestive Health

Digestive health can profoundly influence overall well-being.

- **Dietary Fiber**: Consuming a diet rich in fiber promotes regular bowel movements and aids in preventing digestive disorders.
- **Exercise Benefit**: Regular movement can enhance intestinal muscle contractions, facilitating smoother digestion and preventing constipation.

6. Bone Health and Muscle Mass Maintenance

A synergistic approach is vital to maintain bone density and muscle mass, especially as we age.

- **Dietary Calcium and Vitamin D**: These nutrients are vital for bone health. Sources include dairy products, fortified foods, and sunlight exposure for vitamin D.
- **Weight-bearing Exercises**: Activities like walking, weight lifting, or even yoga can stimulate bone formation and muscle growth, counteracting age-related decline.

7. Cognitive Benefits and Mental Well-being

A combination of a balanced diet and regular exercise can offer cognitive benefits and enhance mental well-being.

- **Brain-boosting Nutrients**: Omega-3 fatty acids, antioxidants, and B vitamins, among others, have been linked to improved brain function and reduced risk of cognitive decline.
- **Exercise and Mental Health**: Regular activity releases endorphins, the body's natural mood elevators. Additionally, exercise has been shown to reduce symptoms of depression, anxiety, and stress.

Conclusion

While diet and exercise are potent longevity-enhancing tools on their own, together they create a symbiotic relationship, each amplifying the benefits of the other. Recognizing and leveraging this synergy can pave the way for a life that's not just longer, but richer in quality, vitality, and joy.

Mental and emotional well-being: the role of diet

Diet plays a crucial role in shaping our physical health, but its impact doesn't stop there. Emerging research suggests that what we eat can profoundly influence our mental and emotional well-being. This intricate relationship between food and mood offers insights into how dietary choices can be utilized to bolster psychological health, thus adding another dimension to our pursuit of longevity.

1. Gut-Brain Connection

The gut and brain, two seemingly disparate organs, are intimately connected. This gut-brain axis facilitates a two-way communication, and the health of one can influence the other.

- **Microbiota's Role**: The gut is home to trillions of microbes. These microbes produce neurotransmitters, like serotonin and dopamine, which regulate mood and emotions. A balanced gut microbiota, fostered by a diet rich in probiotics and fiber, can thus promote emotional well-being.

- **Reducing Inflammation**: Diets high in processed foods can lead to gut inflammation, which, in turn, can trigger brain inflammation and mood disorders. Choosing anti-inflammatory foods can combat this risk.

2. Nutrients and Neurotransmitters

Specific nutrients are precursors to neurotransmitters, the chemical messengers in our brain that regulate mood, stress response, and more.

- **Tryptophan and Serotonin**: Tryptophan, an amino acid found in foods like turkey, eggs, and seeds, is a precursor to serotonin, often dubbed the "happiness hormone." Ensuring adequate tryptophan intake can support optimal serotonin levels.

- **Omega-3 Fatty Acids**: Found abundantly in fatty fish, walnuts, and flaxseeds, omega-3s play a role in dopamine and serotonin production, both crucial for mood stabilization.

3. Blood Sugar and Mood Stability

Blood sugar fluctuations can lead to mood swings, irritability, and fatigue.

- **Complex Carbohydrates**: These are digested slowly, ensuring a steady release of glucose. Foods like whole grains, beans, and vegetables can thus foster mood stability.

- **Avoiding Sugar Spikes**: Diets high in refined sugars can cause rapid glucose spikes and crashes, leading to mood fluctuations. Opting for low-glycemic foods can mitigate this.

4. Vitamins and Cognitive Health

Certain vitamins play a critical role in cognitive function and mental clarity.

- **B Vitamins:** Essential for brain health, deficiencies in B vitamins, especially B12, B6, and folate, can lead to depression and cognitive decline. Leafy greens, legumes, and whole grains are rich sources.
- **Antioxidants:** Vitamins C and E, found in fruits and vegetables, combat oxidative stress, which can negatively impact brain health.

5. Hydration and Brain Function

Even slight dehydration can impair concentration, memory, and mood. Ensuring adequate fluid intake, primarily through water, supports optimal brain function.

6. The Impact of Caffeine

While caffeine can enhance alertness and mood in the short term, excessive intake can lead to anxiety, insomnia, and mood swings. Moderation and individual tolerance are key.

7. Emotional Eating and its Pitfalls

Emotional eating, or using food as a coping mechanism, can lead to a vicious cycle of mood fluctuations and unhealthy dietary patterns. Recognizing these patterns and seeking healthier coping mechanisms is crucial.

Conclusion

The profound connection between diet and emotional well-being offers yet another compelling reason to make conscious dietary choices. By recognizing and harnessing this relationship, we can foster not just physical longevity but a life imbued with mental clarity, emotional balance, and joy. As the adage goes, "You are what you eat," and this couldn't be truer when considering the broader spectrum of holistic well-being.

Holistic approaches to longevity: combining diet, exercise, and mindfulness

The pursuit of longevity extends beyond simply counting the years we live. It's about the quality of those years: vibrant health, mental clarity, and a profound sense of well-being. To achieve this enriched state of life, a holistic approach that integrates diet, exercise, and mindfulness is paramount. Each component, while impactful on its own, becomes exponentially potent when synergistically combined with the others.

1. Diet: The Foundation of Health

- **Nourishing the Body**: A balanced diet provides essential nutrients that fuel the body, support cellular health, and combat inflammation—a key factor in aging and disease.
- **Supporting Mental Health**: As discussed earlier, certain nutrients have a direct impact on neurotransmitter production, influencing mood, stress response, and overall mental well-being.
- **Detoxification**: A clean diet, abundant in antioxidants, aids the body in neutralizing and eliminating toxins, which can accumulate and contribute to degenerative diseases.

2. Exercise: The Pillar of Physical and Cognitive Vitality

- **Cardiovascular Health**: Regular physical activity strengthens the heart, improves blood circulation, and reduces the risk of heart disease. Cardiovascular fitness has been directly linked to longevity.
- **Musculoskeletal Benefits**: Strength training preserves muscle mass and bone density, countering the natural decline that occurs with age. This not only promotes physical independence but also aids in metabolic health.
- **Cognitive Protection**: Exercise stimulates the release of neurotrophic factors, molecules that support brain health, enhance memory, and protect against neurodegenerative diseases.

- **Mood Enhancement**: Physical activity is a natural mood booster. It triggers the release of endorphins, the body's feel-good hormones, combating stress, anxiety, and depression.

3. Mindfulness: The Key to Emotional and Psychological Equilibrium

- **Stress Reduction**: Chronic stress is a silent ager, contributing to inflammation, hormonal imbalances, and a host of chronic conditions. Mindfulness practices, like meditation, have been shown to reduce cortisol levels and mitigate the physiological effects of stress.

- **Emotional Resilience**: Regular mindfulness practice cultivates a heightened awareness of one's emotions, fostering emotional intelligence and resilience. This translates to better coping mechanisms, reduced reactivity, and a balanced mental state.

- **Enhanced Cognitive Function**: Mindfulness can bolster cognitive functions like attention, memory, and problem-solving. Furthermore, practices like meditation may slow age-related cognitive decline.

4. The Synergy of the Triad

- **Reinforcing Benefits**: A nutritious diet can enhance the benefits derived from exercise by fueling workouts and aiding recovery. Similarly, mindfulness practices can amplify the mental benefits of a wholesome diet, creating a positive feedback loop.

- **Comprehensive Well-being**: The combination of diet, exercise, and mindfulness addresses all facets of well-being—physical, mental, emotional, and spiritual. This holistic approach ensures that no aspect of health is neglected.

- **Lifestyle Integration**: By weaving these practices into daily life, they become ingrained habits rather than isolated activities. This ensures sustainability and promotes a life-long commitment to holistic health.

Conclusion

Longevity is a multifaceted gem, reflecting physical vigor, mental acuity, emotional depth, and spiritual growth. By adopting a holistic approach that seamlessly integrates diet, exercise, and mindfulness, one can truly harness the full spectrum of life's potential. As the boundaries between these practices blur, they coalesce into a singular, powerful force, propelling individuals toward a life that is not just long in years, but rich in experiences, insights, and vitality.

Chapter 12: Personalizing Your Dietary Approach

Recognizing individual differences in dietary needs and responses

In the realm of nutrition and health, a one-size-fits-all approach is not only limiting but can also be counterproductive. As our understanding of genetics, metabolism, and individual variances has evolved, so has the appreciation for personalized nutrition. Recognizing and honoring individual differences in dietary needs and responses is paramount for optimal health outcomes.

1. Genetic Factors

- **Metabolic Variability:** Every individual possesses a unique genetic makeup, which can affect the rate and efficiency of metabolism. This can influence how one processes and utilizes nutrients from food.

- **Predisposition to Conditions:** Genetic factors can predispose individuals to certain conditions like lactose intolerance, celiac disease, or a higher likelihood of developing chronic diseases. A tailored diet can help in mitigating these risks.

- **Nutrient Absorption:** Genes can also influence how effectively one absorbs and utilizes certain nutrients, like iron or vitamin D. Recognizing these nuances can guide specific dietary choices.

2. Cultural and Ethnic Considerations

- **Traditional Dietary Patterns:** Different cultures have dietary patterns that have evolved over millennia. These diets are often in sync with the local environment and the genetic makeup of the population.

- **Taste Preferences and Food Values**: Cultural influences shape our taste preferences and the significance we attach to certain foods. It's essential to integrate these preferences while ensuring nutritional adequacy.
- **Metabolic Adaptations**: Over generations, populations might develop specific metabolic adaptations to their traditional diets, affecting nutrient utilization and health outcomes.

3. Age and Life Stages

- **Changing Nutrient Needs**: As we transition through different life stages, from infancy to old age, our nutritional needs change. Tailoring the diet to these changing needs can support growth, development, and optimal health at every stage.
- **Hormonal Influences**: Hormonal changes during life stages like puberty, pregnancy, and menopause can influence dietary needs and how the body responds to certain foods.

4. Personal Health Status and Conditions

- **Disease Management**: Individuals with chronic conditions like diabetes or heart disease often require specialized diets to manage their health and reduce symptoms.
- **Digestive Health Considerations**: Conditions like Irritable Bowel Syndrome (IBS) or Inflammatory Bowel Disease (IBD) can dictate specific dietary choices to manage symptoms and promote gut health.
- **Allergies and Intolerances**: Recognizing and accommodating food allergies and intolerances is crucial for well-being and can significantly affect dietary choices.

5. Lifestyle and Activity Levels

- **Energy Expenditure**: Active individuals and athletes might have elevated caloric and protein needs compared to sedentary individuals. Recognizing these differences can prevent deficiencies and support performance.

- **Occupational Demands**: Some professions might expose individuals to toxins or require heightened mental focus. Tailoring the diet to support detoxification or cognitive function can be beneficial in such cases.

6. Personal Preferences and Philosophies

- **Ethical Choices**: Many individuals choose diets based on ethical beliefs, like veganism. Recognizing and respecting these choices, while ensuring nutritional balance, is vital.

- **Mind-Body Beliefs**: Some dietary choices stem from spiritual or philosophical beliefs about the mind-body connection, like Ayurveda or Traditional Chinese Medicine.

Conclusion

The journey to optimal health is deeply personal. By recognizing the myriad of factors that influence individual dietary needs and responses, we can craft a nutrition plan that not only nourishes the body but also resonates with one's beliefs, preferences, and unique physiological makeup. Personalized nutrition is not just a trend; it's a holistic approach that celebrates individuality in the quest for well-being.

Tips for experimentation and finding what works for each individual

The journey to personalized nutrition is akin to self-discovery. While scientific research, traditional wisdom, and general guidelines provide a solid foundation, at the heart of individualized nutrition lies self-experimentation. Every individual's body is a unique ecosystem, responding differently to various foods, nutrients, and dietary patterns. Discovering what optimally supports your health, energy, and well-being can be empowering. Here are some tips to navigate this exploration with confidence.

1. Start with a Journal

- **Track Everything:** Begin by recording everything you eat, noting the time, quantity, and any immediate reactions you perceive. Over time, patterns will emerge, showing correlations between certain foods and energy levels, mood, digestion, and other physiological responses.

- **Document Physical and Emotional Responses:** Beyond just listing the foods, make a note of how they make you feel. Do certain foods give you energy, or do they make you feel sluggish? Are there foods that uplift your mood or those that cause emotional downturns?

2. Eliminate and Reintroduce

- **Begin with a Clean Slate:** If you suspect certain foods might be causing adverse reactions, eliminate them for a period (usually 2-4 weeks). Common culprits include dairy, gluten, sugar, or specific allergens.

- **Reintroduce Gradually:** After the elimination phase, reintroduce foods one at a time, noting any changes in your body. This step-by-step approach can help pinpoint foods that might be problematic for you.

3. Understand Portion Sizes

- **Don't Overdo It:** Even healthy foods can cause adverse reactions when consumed in large amounts. Understanding portion sizes and moderating intake can help in determining the right balance for your body.

- **Listen to Your Body:** Your body often gives cues about hunger and fullness. Pay attention to these signals and adjust portion sizes accordingly.

4. Seek Professional Guidance

- **Consult a Nutritionist:** If you're unsure where to start or how to interpret the patterns you observe, consulting a nutritionist can be invaluable. They can provide expertise, recommend tests, and guide your experimentation process.

- **Genetic Testing**: Modern advancements allow for genetic testing that can reveal predispositions to certain intolerances or optimized diets based on your DNA. While they don't provide the entire picture, they can be a useful tool in your personalization journey.

5. Embrace Diversity

- **Rotate Foods**: Consuming a wide variety of foods can prevent overexposure to certain compounds and provide a broad spectrum of nutrients. It can also prevent the development of sensitivities due to repetitive consumption.
- **Try New Foods and Cuisines**: Every culture has a rich dietary tradition. Experimenting with foods from different cultures can introduce you to beneficial ingredients and preparation methods.

6. Listen to Your Body

- **Tune In**: Often, our bodies communicate clearly. It's about tuning in and listening. How do you feel after consuming certain foods? Energetic, bloated, refreshed, or lethargic?
- **Trust Your Intuition**: Beyond the physical reactions, trust your instincts. Sometimes, you might feel a natural aversion to or preference for certain foods. These can be cues from your body.

7. Stay Flexible

- **Dietary Needs Change**: As you age, or as life circumstances change (like pregnancy, stress, or physical activity changes), your dietary needs might shift. It's essential to remain adaptable and adjust your diet accordingly.

Conclusion

Embarking on the path of dietary self-experimentation can be both exciting and enlightening. It's about forging a deeper connection with yourself, understanding your unique needs, and nurturing your body in the most personalized way. As you tread this path, remember to be patient, observant, and open-minded, knowing that the journey is as rewarding as the destination.

Emphasizing the importance of listening to one's body

In a world inundated with dietary advice, trends, and ever-evolving research, one of the most profound and timeless pieces of advice remains: listen to your body. While nutritional science offers invaluable insights and generalized guidelines, it's essential to recognize that every individual is unique. Our genes, metabolism, lifestyle, and even gut microbiota differ, meaning what works for one person might not work for another. Thus, attuning to the signals of your own body can guide you in making the best dietary choices for yourself.

1. The Wisdom of the Body

Our bodies are intricate systems with complex feedback mechanisms. They constantly communicate through subtle cues, signaling if something is beneficial or harmful. Over time, humans have become increasingly disconnected from these signals, often due to external influences and distractions. Reconnecting with this innate wisdom is key.

For instance, feeling energetic and focused after a meal can indicate that the foods consumed are well-tolerated and beneficial. On the other hand, feelings of lethargy, bloating, or mood fluctuations can be signs of intolerance or imbalance.

2. Hunger and Fullness Cues

One of the foundational aspects of listening to your body is recognizing genuine hunger and fullness cues.

- **Hunger**: It's not just about the stomach growling. Sometimes, hunger manifests as a dip in energy, difficulty concentrating, or mood shifts. Recognizing and responding to genuine hunger, as opposed to eating out of habit or emotion, can help maintain optimal energy and metabolic balance.

- **Fullness**: Overeating can strain the digestive system and lead to energy imbalances. By paying attention to satiety signals, one can gauge when to stop eating. It's about feeling satisfied, not stuffed.

3. Cravings and Their Underlying Messages

Cravings are often misunderstood. While sometimes they can be driven by emotional needs or habits, other times they might signal nutrient deficiencies or imbalances. For example:

- A craving for chocolate might indicate a magnesium deficiency.
- Desiring salty foods could signal a need for minerals or hydration.

By examining and understanding these cravings, one can address the underlying needs more effectively.

4. The Role of Emotions in Eating

It's vital to differentiate between emotional hunger and physical hunger. Emotional eating can mask as hunger, leading to overconsumption or the intake of foods that might not be nutritionally beneficial. By tuning into emotional states and recognizing patterns, individuals can develop healthier coping mechanisms.

5. Physical Reactions as Feedback

Some reactions are immediate and evident, such as an upset stomach after consuming dairy by lactose-intolerant individuals. Other responses, like breakouts, joint pain, or mood shifts, might be delayed, appearing hours or even days after consuming a trigger food. Documenting and observing these patterns can help in identifying foods or ingredients that might not be suitable for one's unique constitution.

6. Intuition and Mindful Eating

Beyond the tangible cues, there's an element of intuition. Mindful eating, which involves being fully present during meals, can enhance the connection between the body and food. It encourages savoring each bite, appreciating the flavors, and observing how different foods make you feel.

Conclusion

In the quest for optimal health and longevity, external knowledge and guidelines serve as valuable roadmaps. However, the journey is deeply personal. By emphasizing the importance of listening to one's body, individuals can navigate their path with greater clarity and confidence. Remember, your body is your most enduring home. Treat it with care, respect its signals, and it will reciprocate with vitality and well-being.

Chapter 13: Conclusion

The ever-evolving understanding of diet and longevity

As we come to the close of our exploration of diet and its profound influence on lifespan, it's essential to recognize one foundational truth: our understanding is always evolving. Like any scientific field, nutrition and longevity research are dynamic, influenced by new findings, technologies, and shifting global health patterns. The diets and practices that have been elaborated on in this book offer valuable insights based on current knowledge, but the journey of understanding does not end here.

1. A Historical Perspective

Looking back at the annals of history, dietary guidelines have shifted multiple times. Foods once deemed as health elixirs have been relegated to the 'avoid' list and vice versa. Margarine, once promoted as a heart-healthy alternative to butter, later fell from grace due to its trans fats. Eggs, initially chastised for their cholesterol content, have since been vindicated as nutrient powerhouses. These shifts are not a mark of inconsistency but rather a testament to the evolving nature of research and understanding.

2. The Role of Technology and Research

With advancements in technology, especially in areas like genetics, metabolomics, and gut microbiota analysis, we're gaining a more profound and nuanced understanding of how diet affects us. As we develop more sophisticated tools and methodologies, we can expect even more precise and individualized dietary recommendations.

For instance, the Human Genome Project and subsequent advances in genetic testing have ushered in the era of personalized medicine. We're just scratching the surface of understanding how our genes interact with dietary components, and how we can tailor nutrition based on genetic makeup for optimal health outcomes.

3. The Global Landscape

As globalization intensifies, diets are becoming increasingly homogenized. The Western diet, rich in processed foods and high in sugars and unhealthy fats, has been exported around the world. This shift has brought about significant health challenges. However, it has also provided a broader canvas for research. Comparing health outcomes and dietary patterns across diverse populations can yield invaluable insights into the nexus of diet and longevity.

4. Recognizing the Bigger Picture

While diet plays an undeniably pivotal role in health and longevity, it's only one piece of the puzzle. Factors like physical activity, mental well-being, environmental exposures, and social determinants of health interplay with diet to shape our health trajectories. As we move forward, a holistic, integrated approach to longevity will become even more crucial.

5. The Journey of Self-Discovery

As much as we lean on scientific research for guidance, the journey of dietary choices remains deeply personal. As highlighted in previous chapters, listening to one's body and being open to experimentation can lead to the best outcomes. What nourishes one person might not serve another in the same way. Being attuned to one's unique needs, preferences, and reactions is as essential as following broad dietary guidelines.

Conclusion

Our quest for understanding the relationship between diet and longevity is a journey, not a destination. As new research emerges, guidelines will adapt, and recommendations may shift. However, the central tenet remains unchanged: a balanced, varied, and mindful approach to eating, grounded in whole foods and natural ingredients, offers the best promise for a long, healthy life.

While the future holds new discoveries and insights, the age-old wisdom of eating with mindfulness, savoring natural flavors, and respecting the body's signals stands firm. Here's to a life rich in flavor, nourishment, and vitality!

The balance of staying informed while also recognizing individual needs

In our quest for health and longevity, it's tempting to search for definitive answers. With countless diets and a constant stream of new research, the nutrition landscape can be overwhelming. While science offers valuable guidelines, achieving optimal health requires balancing this information with an understanding of our unique physiological and psychological needs. This balance is the cornerstone of a holistic, sustainable approach to health and well-being.

1. The Dynamic World of Nutrition Research

Nutrition science is a rapidly evolving field. Almost every week, there seems to be a new study proclaiming the benefits of a specific food or warning against another. The media often amplifies these findings, sometimes without the nuanced context that's crucial for interpretation. While staying abreast of the latest research is vital, it's equally important to recognize the bigger picture. Individual studies are pieces of a larger puzzle, and it's essential to consider the totality of evidence rather than reacting to each new piece in isolation.

2. Individual Variability: One Size Doesn't Fit All

Even with a comprehensive understanding of nutritional science, there's no universally perfect diet. Genetic makeup, gut microbiota, lifestyle factors, and even individual preferences play a role in determining the ideal dietary approach for each person. What works wonders for one might be detrimental for another. The concept of bio-individuality — the idea that each of us has unique food and lifestyle needs — underscores the importance of personalizing our approach to diet.

3. Navigating Information Overload

With easy access to information, it's common to encounter conflicting advice. One day, a certain food is touted as a 'superfood,' and the next, it's linked to potential health concerns. Such contradictions can be confusing. To navigate this maze, it's helpful to:

- **Critical Analysis:** Examine the source of information. Peer-reviewed studies offer more reliable insights than anecdotal claims.
- **Holistic View:** Instead of fixating on individual foods, focus on overall dietary patterns and lifestyle.
- **Consult Professionals:** Registered dietitians or nutritionists can provide personalized advice grounded in solid research.

4. Tuning into Intuitive Eating

While science and research are invaluable, tuning into our body's signals is equally crucial. Intuitive eating, a practice that encourages listening to internal cues (like hunger and fullness) rather than external rules, can be a game-changer. By fostering a deep connection with our bodies and recognizing how different foods make us feel, we can make informed choices that align with both scientific guidance and personal well-being.

5. The Mental Aspect of Diet

Mental well-being is intrinsically linked with diet. Obsessing over every dietary choice or experiencing guilt over 'indulgences' can be counter-productive. A balanced approach recognizes that while nutrition is vital, occasional deviations from the 'ideal' diet won't derail health goals. Flexibility, kindness towards oneself, and recognizing the broader context of life's pleasures can enhance both mental health and overall well-being.

Conclusion

Achieving the balance between staying informed and recognizing individual needs is more art than science. It requires a dance between external knowledge and internal wisdom. As we close this exploration into diet and longevity, remember that the journey to optimal health isn't a linear path defined by strict rules. Instead, it's a dynamic process of learning, adapting, and most importantly, listening — to both the wisdom of science and the wisdom of our own bodies. In this balance lies the true essence of holistic health and longevity.

Encouragement for readers to take proactive steps towards healthier dietary choices

The journey of understanding the intricate relationship between diet and longevity has been enlightening, to say the least. From the ancient wisdom of the Mediterranean diet to the cutting-edge science of caloric restriction, it's evident that the choices we make at the dining table play a significant role in our health and lifespan. But understanding these principles is only half the battle. The real challenge, and opportunity, lies in putting this knowledge into action. In this closing section, we offer words of encouragement and guidance to empower you to take proactive steps towards healthier dietary choices.

1. Every Step Counts

Embracing healthier dietary choices isn't about perfection; it's about progression. Whether you're considering a switch to a plant-based diet or merely aiming to reduce your sugar intake, every positive step you take has the potential to improve your health. Small, consistent changes often lead to lasting results. Don't be daunted by the idea of overhauling your entire diet overnight. Start with one change, master it, and then build from there.

2. Celebrate the Journey, Not Just the Destination

While the ultimate goal might be to achieve optimal health and longevity, it's essential to find joy in the journey. Celebrate the new flavors you discover, the energy spikes from a healthier meal, or even the sense of accomplishment from cooking a nutritious dish at home. These moments of joy not only make the journey enjoyable but also motivate you to stay on the path.

3. Seek Support

Change, especially when it comes to deeply ingrained eating habits, can be challenging. Surrounding yourself with supportive friends, family, or communities can make a world of difference. Whether it's a buddy who joins you in trying a new diet or an online community where you can share recipes and experiences, having a support system can be the wind beneath your wings.

4. Stay Informed, But Trust Yourself

While it's crucial to stay updated with the latest in nutrition science, remember that you are the expert of your own body. Listen to it. If a particular diet or food doesn't agree with you, it's okay to trust your experience and make adjustments. Marrying external knowledge with internal awareness creates a powerful synergy for optimal health.

5. Revisit and Re-evaluate

As you progress on this journey, take time to revisit and re-evaluate your dietary choices. What worked wonderfully at one stage of life might need tweaking as circumstances change. Regular check-ins with yourself, and possibly with a nutrition professional, can ensure that you remain aligned with your health goals.

6. Keep the Big Picture in Mind

While diet is a significant pillar of health, it's just one piece of the puzzle. Adequate sleep, regular exercise, mental well-being, and strong social connections are equally crucial. Embrace a holistic view of health where dietary choices complement other lifestyle factors.

Final Words

As we conclude this exploration, remember that the path to longevity is a marathon, not a sprint. It's about making informed choices, listening to your body, and enjoying the myriad experiences that come with living a full, healthy life. Armed with knowledge, support, and a dash of determination, you're well-equipped to make dietary choices that serve not just your body, but also your soul. Here's to a life of vitality, joy, and countless delicious, nutritious meals!

Appendix A: Glossary of terms

This glossary provides brief explanations of some of the key terms and concepts mentioned throughout the book. It serves as a quick reference for readers seeking clarity on specific terms.

1. Antioxidants

Substances that can prevent or slow damage to cells caused by free radicals. They are commonly found in fruits, vegetables, and certain types of tea.

2. Caloric Restriction (CR)

A dietary regimen that reduces calorie intake without incurring malnutrition. CR has been shown in some studies to increase lifespan in various organisms.

3. Carbohydrates

One of the primary macronutrients, carbohydrates are organic compounds that include sugars, starches, and cellulose. They are a primary source of energy for the body.

4. Essential Nutrients

Nutrients required for normal physiological function that the body cannot synthesize on its own. They must be obtained from dietary sources.

5. Healthspan

The portion of a person's life during which they are in good health and free from chronic diseases. It's different from lifespan, which is the total length of one's life.

6. Intermittent Fasting (IF)

An eating pattern that cycles between periods of eating and fasting. It doesn't prescribe what foods to eat but rather when you should eat.

7. Ketosis

A metabolic state wherein the body burns fat for fuel in the absence of carbohydrates. It's the foundational principle behind the ketogenic diet.

8. Macronutrients

The primary nutrients the body needs in large amounts: carbohydrates, proteins, and fats.

9. Micronutrients

Nutrients the body needs in smaller amounts, such as vitamins and minerals.

10. Omega-3 Fatty Acids

A type of polyunsaturated fat that's linked to several health benefits. Commonly found in fatty fish, walnuts, and flaxseeds.

11. Phytonutrients

Natural chemicals or compounds produced by plants. They can have health-promoting properties including antioxidant effects.

12. Processed Foods

Foods that have been modified from their natural state through various methods, often to extend shelf life or enhance flavor. They often contain added sugars, salt, and unhealthy fats.

13. Probiotics

Live bacteria and yeasts that are beneficial for the digestive system. They can be found in fermented foods and certain dietary supplements.

14. Protein

One of the primary macronutrients, proteins are made up of amino acids and play many critical roles in the body. Sources include meat, dairy, and legumes.

15. Vegan Diet

A diet that excludes all animal products, including meat, dairy, and eggs. It relies solely on plant-based foods.

16. Vegetarian Diet

A diet that excludes certain animal products. There are various forms of vegetarianism, with some vegetarians choosing to eat dairy or eggs, but not meat.

17. Vitamins

Organic molecules that are vital micronutrients required in small quantities for essential metabolic reactions in the body.

18. Whole Foods

Foods that are not processed or refined and are free from additives or other artificial substances. Examples include fresh fruits, vegetables, and grains.

19. Blue Zones

Regions in the world where people live much longer than average. These zones are known for their unique dietary and lifestyle habits.

20. Glycemic Index (GI)

A measure of how quickly and by how much a food raises blood sugar levels. Foods with a low GI are slower to raise blood sugar levels compared to foods with a high GI.

By familiarizing oneself with these terms, one can better understand the complexities of nutrition and its impact on overall health and longevity.

Appendix B: Recommended reading and resources

Navigating the world of nutrition and longevity can be challenging, given the vast amount of information available. To assist you in your journey, here's a curated list of books, articles, and online resources that delve deeper into the topics discussed in this book.

1. Books

- "The Blue Zones" by Dan Buettner

An exploration of the five places in the world where people live the longest, healthiest lives. Buettner provides insights into the dietary, lifestyle, and societal factors that contribute to longevity in these regions.

- "How Not to Die" by Dr. Michael Greger

A comprehensive look at the role of diet in preventing, arresting, and reversing many of our leading causes of death and disability.

- "The Longevity Diet" by Dr. Valter Longo

Dr. Longo, a leading expert on longevity, presents a unique combination of the Mediterranean and Okinawan diets. The book is backed by extensive research on how to live a longer, healthier life.

- "Eat to Live" by Dr. Joel Fuhrman

This book delves deep into nutrient-rich eating and its transformative power, offering a detailed diet plan that can lead to sustained weight loss and overall improved health.

2. Articles

- **"The Role of Diet and Exercise in the Transgenerational Epigenetic Landscape of T2DM"** published in *Nature Reviews Endocrinology*

A deep dive into how our dietary and exercise habits can impact not only our health but that of future generations.

- **"Effects of Intermittent Fasting on Health, Aging, and Disease"** published in *The New England Journal of Medicine*

This article offers a comprehensive review of the current science behind intermittent fasting and its potential benefits.

3. Websites & Online Resources

- **https://nutritionfacts.org**

A non-commercial, science-based source that provides the latest research on nutrition. Dr. Michael Greger and his team review various nutrition-related research articles and present them in easy-to-understand videos and articles.

- **https://www.bluezones.com**

This website expands on Dan Buettner's work and provides more insights, stories, and tips from the Blue Zones regions.

- **http://www.whfoods.com**

An exhaustive resource providing detailed information on various foods, their nutrient content, and their health benefits.

4. Podcasts

- **"The Nutrition Diva's Quick and Dirty Tips for Eating Well and Feeling Fabulous"**

Monica Reinagel provides brief, informative episodes on various nutrition topics, debunking myths and offering practical advice.

- "FoundMyFitness" with Dr. Rhonda Patrick

Dr. Patrick delves deep into various health topics, often with a focus on the molecular mechanisms behind dietary and lifestyle interventions.

5. Apps

- MyFitnessPal

A comprehensive app for tracking diet and exercise, it has a vast database of foods and can help users understand their macro and micronutrient intake.

- Zero-Fasting Tracker

For those interested in intermittent fasting, this app provides tracking tools, tips, and reminders to help maintain fasting schedules.

By delving into these recommended resources, you can further your understanding and appreciation of the intricate relationship between diet, health, and longevity. As with any topic, it's crucial to approach it with an open mind and a critical eye, ensuring you gather information from reputable sources and remain adaptable as the science evolves.

Appendix C: Sample meal plans and recipes for each diet type

Navigating the intricacies of various diet types can be challenging, but having a few sample meal plans and recipes at your fingertips can provide a helpful starting point. Below are sample meal plans for a day on each diet, along with a suggested recipe.

1. Mediterranean Diet

Sample Meal Plan:

- **Breakfast:** Greek yogurt with honey, almonds, and fresh berries.
- **Lunch:** Grilled chicken salad with olives, feta, tomatoes, cucumbers, and a lemon-oregano vinaigrette.
- **Dinner:** Baked salmon with a side of quinoa, steamed broccoli, and a drizzle of olive oil.

Recipe – Mediterranean Chickpea Salad:

- Ingredients: Canned chickpeas, sliced cucumber, cherry tomatoes, red onion, feta cheese, olive oil, lemon juice, oregano.
- Method: Mix all ingredients in a bowl. Season with salt and pepper.

2. Vegan Diet

Sample Meal Plan:

- **Breakfast:** Smoothie with spinach, almond milk, banana, chia seeds, and a scoop of plant-based protein powder.
- **Lunch:** Vegan wrap with hummus, avocado, lettuce, tomato, and roasted red pepper.
- **Dinner:** Vegan stir-fry with tofu, broccoli, bell peppers, zucchini, and a soy-ginger sauce over brown rice.

Recipe – Vegan Lentil Soup:

- Ingredients: Lentils, vegetable broth, diced tomatoes, carrots, onions, celery, garlic, cumin, turmeric, spinach.
- Method: Sauté vegetables, add lentils and broth. Cook until lentils are tender. Add spinach at the end.

3. Paleo Diet

Sample Meal Plan:

- **Breakfast:** Scrambled eggs with spinach and avocado.
- **Lunch:** Salad with grilled steak, mixed greens, cherry tomatoes, and a vinaigrette.
- **Dinner:** Roast chicken with steamed asparagus and sautéed mushrooms.

Recipe – Paleo Spaghetti Squash and Meatballs:

- Ingredients: Spaghetti squash, ground beef or turkey, almond flour, egg, garlic, tomato sauce, basil, oregano.
- Method: Bake spaghetti squash. Mix meat, almond flour, egg, and spices to form meatballs. Bake meatballs. Serve with sauce over squash.

4. Ketogenic Diet

Sample Meal Plan:

- **Breakfast:** Bacon and eggs fried in butter.
- **Lunch:** Spinach and feta stuffed chicken breast with a side of green beans.
- **Dinner:** Zucchini noodles with a creamy avocado-pesto sauce and shrimp.

Recipe – Keto Avocado Chocolate Mousse:

- Ingredients: Avocado, unsweetened cocoa powder, stevia or erythritol, vanilla extract, coconut cream.

- Method: Blend all ingredients until smooth. Chill before serving.

5. Plant-based Whole Foods Diet

Sample Meal Plan:

- **Breakfast:** Oatmeal topped with fresh berries, nuts, and a splash of almond milk.
- **Lunch:** Quinoa salad with roasted vegetables and a tahini dressing.
- **Dinner:** Lentil and vegetable curry over brown rice.

Recipe – Stuffed Bell Peppers:

- Ingredients: Bell peppers, brown rice, black beans, corn, onions, garlic, diced tomatoes, cumin, chili powder.
- Method: Sauté onion and garlic, add beans, corn, rice, tomatoes, and spices. Stuff mixture into bell peppers. Bake until tender.

By incorporating these sample meal plans and recipes into your routine, you can kickstart your journey on any of these diets. Remember, variety is key – feel free to adapt and modify these plans to suit your preferences and nutritional needs.